BOOK REVIEWS

'If you are a smoker who has tried and failed to quit, this book could be for you. Over the past decade in the UK, vaping has emerged as the most popular means to quit smoking, and one of the most effective. Vaping is controversial but can save smokers' lives. This book deals with those controversies head on, and explains why, despite uncertainties over long term harms and other possible unwanted effects, vaping is one of the most powerful tools now available to help smokers quit. So, if you are a smoker, and especially a smoker who hasn't tried vaping, read this book, and try it now.'

Emeritus Professor John Britton.
Epidemiologist and former consultant in respiratory medicine, University of Nottingham, UK; and Former Chair, Tobacco Advisory Group, Royal College of Physicians (UK)

'This book is a must for any smoker who wants to know if vaping can help them quit (I wish I'd known about it earlier). Accurate information on vaping and nicotine is hard to find – even health professionals are not well informed. This book is a valuable resource that is long overdue and will help many smokers finally give up for good.'

Senator Hollie Hughes.
Liberal Senator for New South Wales; Chair of the Australian Senate Select Committee on Tobacco Harm Reduction

'This book is a valuable resource for smokers, doctors and regulators. Smokers will get clear information on the benefits of switching to vaping and some excellent practical guidance on how to do it; doctors will learn about an important topic that is not covered in their education; and politicians and regulators will obtain some clarity about the difference between facts and ideologically motivated misinformation that has been dominating this field. The book has great potential to improve both individual and public health.'

Professor Peter Hajek.
Professor of Clinical Psychology and Director of the Health and Lifestyle Research Unit at the Wolfson Institute of Preventive Medicine, Queen Mary University of London

'Dr Mendelsohn provides an excellent review of vaping and the harm reduction debate. This book provides pragmatic information for the smoker who is thinking about vaping as a way to quit, and for the vaper who would like to learn more about the current state of science on electronic cigarettes.'

Professor Neal Benowitz.
Emeritus Professor of Medicine, Centre for Tobacco Control Research and Education, University of California, San Francisco, USA

'Dr Colin Mendelsohn has written a brilliant book about vaping for tobacco harm reduction. He dispels myths and provides facts and useful information about vaping, including the pros and cons and how to go about it. This book is for smokers, their families and doctors wanting to help smokers quit, and will save many lives.'

Dr Joe Kosterich.
General practitioner and health industry consultant; Chairman, Australian Tobacco Harm Reduction Association

'Colin Mendelsohn has written a very informative book on nicotine vaping for smokers and general practitioners. He clearly explains what vaping is, the varieties of devices that can be used, how they can be legally obtained, and how smokers can use them for smoking cessation, or as lower risk ways of obtaining nicotine. He corrects common misconceptions about the comparative risks of smoking and vaping and provides an invaluable resource for GPs to advise smokers on the pros and cons of vaping versus smoking and on using vaping to quit smoking.'

Emeritus Professor Wayne Hall.
Centre for Youth Substance Abuse Research at the University of Queensland; Visiting Professor at the London School of Hygiene and Tropical Medicine

'This book provides a simple and concise overview of the evidence on e-cigarettes and practical advice for smokers, and health professionals, who want to know more about the use of e-cigarettes as a route out of smoking tobacco. This is likely to be especially helpful for those who have tried and failed with conventional smoking cessation aids.'

Professor Hayden McRobbie.
National Drug and Alcohol Research Centre, University of New South Wales, Sydney

'This book written by Dr Mendelsohn is a must-read for all smokers who want to quit. Easy to read and based on scientific information, the book spans the full 360 degrees of the world of vaping. Consumers, policymakers, health professionals will find it insightful. Many will finally understand the value of switching to e-cigarettes as a far less harmful alternative to smoking tobacco.'

Professor Riccardo Polosa.
Professor of Internal Medicine and Respiratory Physician, University of Catania, Italy; Founder of the Center of Excellence for the Acceleration of Harm Reduction (CoEHAR), University of Catania, Italy

'This book is essential reading for policy makers, public health practitioners and – most importantly – people who smoke cigarettes and seek to be empowered to make informed personal health decisions. Dr Mendelsohn presents the evidence for vaping in a clear and readable manner, replacing hysteria with facts and moralism with compassion.'

Adjunct Professor David T. Sweanor JD.
Chair of the Advisory Board, Centre for Health Law, Policy & Ethics, University of Ottawa, Canada; and Adjunct Professor, Faculty of Law, University of Ottawa

STOP SMOKING START VAPING

The Healthy Truth about Vaping

DR COLIN MENDELSOHN

First published in Australia by Aurora House
www.aurorahouse.com.au

This edition published November 2021
Copyright © Colin Mendelsohn 2021

Cover design: Donika Mishineva | www.artofdonika.com
Typesetting and e-book design: Amit Dey

The right of Colin Mendelsohn to be identified as Author of the Work has been asserted in accordance with the Copyright, Designs and Patents Act 1988.

ISBN number: 978-1-922697-12-7 (Paperback)

 A catalogue record for this book is available from the National Library of Australia

Distributed by: Ingram Content: www.ingramcontent.com
Australia: phone +613 9765 4800 |
email lsiaustralia@ingramcontent.com
Milton Keynes UK: phone +44 (0)845 121 4567 |
email enquiries@ingramcontent.com
La Vergne, TN USA: phone +1 800 509 4156 |
email inquiry@lightningsource.com

CONTENTS

CASE STUDIES

DEDICATION

To Australia's three million smokers
and my father and father-in-law, who both died
of cancer from smoking

FOREWORD

I have great pleasure in writing a foreword for this important book which could help prevent the early deaths of possibly hundreds of thousands of Australian smokers.

As a specialist in addiction medicine and the Director of the Alcohol and Drug Service at St Vincents' Hospital in inner Sydney for over thirty years, I have treated many thousands of people who use drugs. I have also been actively involved in drug harm reduction campaigns to reduce the death and disease from drug use. I have campaigned with colleagues for needle and syringe programs to prevent HIV in people who inject drugs, safe injecting rooms, methadone programs and the distribution of condoms to prevent HIV and other sexually transmitted infections. Although fiercely resisted initially, these initiatives have saved countless lives and are now widely accepted.

I see strong parallels with vaping nicotine as a way to reduce the harm from smoking in adult smokers. Most smokers try to quit and fail repeatedly. Tragically, up to two out of three who continue to smoke will die prematurely from their smoking and will live ten years less on average. Clearly additional, effective strategies are needed to help them. Many people who inject heroin also struggle to quit on their own. Some do. But many benefit from help from health professionals including methadone treatment.

When Colin asked me to look into vaping nicotine as a safer alternative for smoking, I could see that this harm reduction strategy had huge potential to help smokers, many of whom are disadvantaged and suffering huge financial stress from highly priced cigarettes.

I have known Colin for over thirty years. He has been dedicated to helping smokers quit during that time and has trained more health professionals on smoking than anyone else in Australia. He has been actively involved in research and publishing scientific articles on smoking.

Colin was the first doctor in Australia to recognise the potential for vaping. He could see how it was helping his patients to quit, often after all other treatments had failed. He studied the evidence and overseas experience and became a passionate advocate for vaping, which was facing widespread opposition from Australian government health departments, medical associations and health charities.

In 2017, along with several colleagues we established the Australian Tobacco Harm Reduction Association, a health promotion charity, to raise awareness of vaping nicotine and to educate the public about it. We have been working closely together on vaping since then.

Vaping nicotine is now Australia's most popular and most effective quitting aid. It allows smokers to get the nicotine they need while still enjoying the smoking ritual and sensations of 'smoking'. Vaping is not risk-free but is a far less harmful alternative to smoking as almost all of the harmful toxins and carcinogens in smoke are absent. Vaping is only for smokers and should not be used by non-smokers of any age.

I am delighted Colin has written this much needed book. He has an encyclopaedic knowledge of the area, is amazingly up to date and completely committed to the scientific evidence. Smokers need accurate information on vaping and it is very hard to access this in Australia due to the entrenched opposition, alarmist media reports and restrictive regulations around vaping. This book provides the latest information in a readable and well-organised way.

If you are a smoker who has been unable to quit with other treatments, this book is for you. It outlines the scientific evidence for vaping and gives practical, step-by-step advice on how to get started with vaping such as what to buy, where to get it and how to use it safely and legally.

The book is also a valuable guide for GPs and other health practitioners who wish to counsel smokers on vaping. It will also be useful to a wide range of other stakeholders as it also addresses the controversies about vaping and how it should be regulated in Australia.

I have seen the enormous public health benefit from other drug harm reduction strategies, and I am convinced that vaping will be even more beneficial. If you are a smoker, switching to vaping will improve your health, expose you to far fewer toxins, save you money and make you feel and smell much better.

Quitting smoking is the best thing you will ever do for your health. If you can't quit smoking, switching to vaping is the next best thing. This book will show you how and could save your life.

Dr Alex Wodak AM
Director, Australian Tobacco Harm Reduction Association
Chair, Australia21
Emeritus Consultant, St Vincents' Hospital, Sydney

WHY I HAVE WRITTEN THIS BOOK

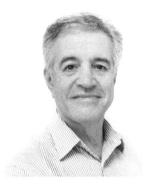

The most rewarding part of general practice for me has been the long-term relationships I developed with patients. I saw people through good and bad times, got to know their families and developed close professional connections. It was heartbreaking when someone I cared about developed a serious illness.

Smoking kills 21,000 Australians every year and most of these deaths are preventable.[1] There is a huge human cost behind the statistics. I can recall many sad stories.

I met John soon after I started my practice. He was a hotel manager who had planned to retire with his wife at the age of sixty-five 'up the coast'. They worked hard, putting money aside for their new lifestyle, and purchased a cottage near the water. John was also a heavy smoker who tried many times to quit, but always seemed to slip back into smoking. John tragically died from a heart attack one week before he was about to move.

Margaret also worked hard all her life as a salesperson and had three daughters. She smoked from the age of eleven and always felt guilty that she couldn't quit, even when pregnant. When she died from lung cancer at the age of sixty, she left a grieving husband and family. She told me her biggest regret was not being able to grow old with her husband and see her grandchildren grow up.

When I was forty, my father also died from cancer due to smoking. Like me, he was a general practitioner and knew well the risk he was taking. He had a long series of illnesses due to smoking but could not quit. He also knew his grandchildren only briefly.

These stories are not unusual. Up to two out of three Australian smokers will die prematurely from their smoking.[2] It soon became obvious to me that the greatest impact I could have as a doctor was to help smokers quit. I have spent over thirty years focussed on smoking, helping smokers quit, teaching health professionals, writing articles and doing research.

However, even with the most effective treatments available and the best care I could provide, most of my smoking patients could not quit. This was incredibly discouraging to patients, but also to me! I was supposed to be the smoking expert (I became known as the 'smoking doctor') and yet I was having far more failures than successes. I clearly needed new and effective treatments.

Vaping nicotine arrived in the United Kingdom and United States in 2006/7 and reports started appearing in Australia over the next few years. Smokers were quitting with this new technology. The early evidence was promising, and I wanted to find out more.

In 2015, I went to London, which was the epicentre of research on vaping at the time. I met with several leading researchers and advocates, Peter Hajek, Clive Bates and Martin Dockrell, who confirmed my impression that vaping had huge potential to help smokers.

When I returned to Australia, I wrote my first article on vaping in the *Medical Journal of Australia* titled, 'Electronic cigarettes: what can we learn from the UK experience?'.[3]

Even in those early days with less effective devices, the results were encouraging. Vaping was not a silver bullet, but it helped many of my smoking patients quit, notably many who had previously failed with all other treatments. Vaping let them continue to enjoy the nicotine they craved and replicated the hand-to-mouth action and sensations of smoking, but with only a small fraction of the toxins in smoke.

Since then, there has been a huge amount of research confirming that vaping nicotine is a more effective quitting aid than nicotine replacement therapy (nicotine patches, gums etc.) and is far less harmful than smoking. Smokers who switch to vaping have significant health improvements, feel and smell better and save thousands of dollars each year.

It is no surprise that vaping is the most popular quitting aid globally. It has been embraced by many governments and leading health and medical organisations around the world. However, in Australia there is widespread opposition to vaping and most smokers think it is equally or more harmful than smoking.

In 2017, several medical colleagues and I established the Australian Tobacco Harm Reduction Association (ATHRA), a health promotion charity, to educate the public and other stakeholders about vaping. We naively thought that sharing the evidence would lead to a change in attitudes and policy. How wrong we were! There are other hidden motives driving the opposition to vaping and these are discussed in Part 3.

We are optimistic that vaping will be accepted as a mainstream quitting aid in time. It will be too late to help John, Margaret or my father, but it has the potential to save the lives of hundreds of thousands of Australian smokers who cannot quit in other ways.

We will look back in twenty years and wonder why we didn't embrace it earlier.

If you are a smoker who can't or doesn't want to quit smoking, this book gives you the information you need to make an informed decision about vaping. It's your decision, but it could be the best decision you ever make.

About me

I was a general practitioner for twenty-seven years with a special focus on smoking and I now work exclusively in tobacco treatment in Sydney, helping smokers to quit.

I was the Founding Chairman of the Australian Tobacco Harm Reduction Association (ATHRA) and have been a vocal advocate for vaping nicotine in Australia. I am also a member of the committee that develops the Royal Australian College of General Practitioners' national smoking cessation guidelines.[4]

I have written many peer-reviewed articles on smoking and vaping in scientific journals and have conducted hundreds of lectures, workshops and seminars for health professionals on smoking and vaping, more than anyone else in Australia.

I was a Conjoint Associate Professor in the School of Public Health and Community Medicine at the University of New South Wales, Sydney from 2016-2019. I am an investigator on a current government-funded (NHMRC) trial on vaping nicotine and have served on the NSW Health advisory committee on e-cigarettes.

I am a member of the Vaping Cessation Expert Panel at the Centre for Addiction and Mental Health (Toronto, Canada), which is developing guidelines for ceasing vaping for the Ontario Ministry of Health. I am also on the Expert Advisory Group for the Coalition of Asia Pacific Tobacco Harm Reduction Association (CAPHRA).

I was previously Vice President of the Australian Association of Smoking Cessation Professionals, Australia's peak body for health professionals who help smokers quit. You can visit my website for more information about me at www.colinmendelsohn.com.au.

Financial disclosure

I have never received funding of any kind from vaping or tobacco companies. No funding has been provided to prepare this book. No brand names or Australian vaping businesses are identified in the book except in the testimonials. I receive no commissions or benefit from the sale of any vaping products.

I have received payments for teaching, consulting and conference expenses from companies that make stop-smoking pharmaceuticals. These are Pfizer Australia, GlaxoSmithKline, Johnson & Johnson Pacific and Perrigo Australia. I am on the Champix Advisory Board of Pfizer Australia.

HOW TO USE THIS BOOK

If you are in a hurry to start vaping, you can begin with the quick-start guide on page xxiii and refer to Part 2 for more detailed advice. I recommend you read as much of Part 2 as you can *before* going to a vape shop to make your purchasing decisions easier.

The book also provides more information and evidence for those who want to do a deep dive into the subject.

Part 1 explains what vaping is and outlines the scientific evidence. Is it safe? Is it an effective quitting aid? Is it legal? How harmful is nicotine? Part 2 is a practical guide to getting started with vaping. What to buy, where to get vaping products and how to use them.

Part 3 explores the controversies about vaping. Why is it opposed by most Australian health and medical authorities? What are the hidden reasons underpinning their objections? How should vaping be regulated in Australia and what can we do to accelerate the uptake of vaping? The Appendix includes a glossary of terms, additional resources and supporting health organisations.

Please read the case studies at the end of each chapter. These are real stories by real people just like you and show how vaping could change your life for the better.

Whether you decide to read a little or a lot, one thing is for certain. If you are a current adult smoker who can't quit, switching to vaping is the best thing you will ever do for your health and your pocket! Be inspired by reading the testimonials from other vapers and give it a try.

I hope this book helps you on your journey to a smoke-free future! Please let me know how you go.

A note to non-Australian readers

This book is also written for you. It provides the evidence for the safety and effectiveness of vaping nicotine and how to make the switch from smoking to this lifesaving alternative. The discussion on why vaping is opposed by some anti-vaping advocates also applies in your country. The book frequently refers to evidence and experiences in other countries. However, there are some small differences to be aware of.

In your country, you can simply purchase nicotine e-liquid as an adult consumer product from vape shops and other retail outlets. In Australia, authorities classify nicotine liquid as a medicine which requires a prescription from a doctor. Australia's complex system of importing nicotine e-liquid and pharmacy purchases do not apply to you.

Be aware that some countries such as the UK and EU set a limit of 20mg/mL nicotine and some different laws and regulations may apply. In particular, the draconian penalties for unauthorised importation or use of nicotine liquid in Australia are not relevant in other western countries.

In many countries, vaping nicotine is a first-line quitting aid and smokers are not required to try other methods first.

Disclaimer

The content of this book is not to be relied upon by anyone using it or reading it as a medical consultation or medical advice. All medical information is general in nature and does not constitute individual clinical advice. Readers of the book should contact their own doctor or other health professional in relation to any clinical concerns you may have.

All patients who have provided case studies have given written consent to be named and identified in the book.

Quick-start guide for smokers

1. Select a simple starter kit

- Visit your local vape shop
- Choose a starter kit that suits your needs, based on similarity to a cigarette, ease of use, size, nicotine delivery, battery capacity and your budget
- Most smokers initially prefer a device suited to 'mouth-to-lung' vaping, which is like smoking
- Pod vapes and vape pens are the most popular starter kits for beginners. Other suitable models are disposables and 'cigalikes'
- More powerful and customisable advanced models are available if preferred
- Ask the vape shop staff to show you how to fill and use the device safely and how to change the pod or coil. Be sure to read the manual
- Buy some spare coils and/or pods if using these

2. Choose an e-liquid

- Consider whether you are nicotine dependent and if you need nicotine
- Select a nicotine concentration to match your nicotine dependence and vaping device
- Select freebase nicotine or nicotine salt, depending on the device and nicotine concentration you are using and personal preference
- Use nicotine salt for higher nicotine concentrations, generally for >20mg/mL
- Most new vapers start with the familiar tobacco flavour and later switch to fruit, dessert or mint flavours

3. Visit your GP

- You need a prescription from a doctor to import, use and possess nicotine legally in Australia
- Your doctor will help you decide whether vaping is appropriate for you
- Ask your GP for further advice and support for your quit attempt

4. Buy your e-liquid

With a prescription, you can legally purchase nicotine e-liquid in two ways:

- Import it from overseas under the Personal Importation Scheme. This can be either
  - o Pre-mixed flavoured nicotine e-liquid in a bottle or pod, or
  - o Concentrated nicotine (100mg/mL) for mixing with flavoured nicotine-free e-liquid purchased locally. This has greater risks and is for careful use by experienced vapers only

  Email or upload a copy of your prescription to the overseas vendor so it can be enclosed with your order

- From a participating Australian (physical or online) pharmacy. This requires a special prescription from an 'Authorised Prescriber' for nicotine (ask if your GP is registered). Pharmacies can
  - o Supply a limited range of commercial nicotine e-liquids in bottles or pods
  - o Prepare nicotine e-liquids from the basic ingredients (compounding pharmacies only)
- If you don't need nicotine, purchase nicotine-free e-liquid from your local vape shop

5. Start vaping

- Take long slow puffs whenever you get the urge to smoke
- A little coughing is common but usually settles
- Don't be afraid to carefully increase the nicotine concentration if needed
- Make sure you vape frequently enough so you are not tempted to smoke
- It is safe to vape and smoke for a while until you are ready to quit smoking
- It is very important to stop smoking completely
- Persevere until you find the combination of device, nicotine concentration and flavour that works for you
- Vape courteously when around others as you do when smoking
- Always keep spare coils, pods, adequate e-liquid supplies and a second charged device available
- Once you have quit smoking, stop vaping if you can, but continue vaping if it is keeping you from relapsing to smoking

6. Vape safely

- Keep nicotine e-liquids in child-resistant containers and out of the reach of children and pets
- Always use gloves when handling high concentrations of nicotine
- Learn about battery safety. Always use the cable that came with your device. Charging in a computer or game console USB port is generally safe. If using mains power, use a low amp (0.5-1amp) wall charging adapter
- If using removable batteries
  - Never carry loose batteries in your pocket or purse without a plastic case
  - Only use reputable brands, use a good quality external charger and discard batteries if damaged

PART 1

The Evidence on Vaping and Nicotine

1

WHAT IS VAPING?

Take-home messages

- In Australia, vaping nicotine is considered a legitimate second-line treatment for smokers who can't quit with conventional treatments
- Vaping delivers nicotine and the smoking ritual, without most of the toxins and carcinogens from burning tobacco
- Vaping is the most popular quitting aid in Australia
- It is more effective than nicotine replacement therapies (nicotine gum, patches etc.)
- The best option for smokers is always to quit smoking and nicotine altogether if you can
- Vaping is on average about 10% of the cost of smoking
- Vaping should NOT be taken up by non-smokers, especially young people who don't smoke

Vaping is a way to quit smoking by getting nicotine and the familiar smoking ritual without the thousands of toxins in cigarette smoke. A vaping device (vaporiser, e-cigarette, vape or ENDS) heats a liquid solution (usually containing nicotine) into an aerosol which is inhaled and exhaled as a visible mist. Vaping replicates the hand-to-mouth habit and sensations of smoking and is a satisfying and less harmful substitute.

In Australia, vaping is considered a second-line quitting aid for adult smokers who are unable or unwilling to quit smoking with other methods.[4] It is appealing to smokers and is the most popular aid for quitting or reducing smoking in Australia[5] and in other western countries such as the United Kingdom,[6] the United States[7] and Europe.[8]

Vaping nicotine is significantly more effective than nicotine replacement therapy (nicotine patch, gum, lozenges, spray).[9] Some smokers use it as a short-term quitting aid, switching to vaping and then ceasing vaping as well, perhaps over three to six months. Others continue to vape long-term to avoid relapsing to smoking.[10]

Vaping is not risk-free but is far less harmful than smoking. Almost all the harm from smoking is from the thousands of toxic chemicals and carcinogens (cancer-causing chemicals) from burning tobacco.[11] Vaporisers do not contain tobacco and there is no combustion or smoke. The UK Royal College of Physicians estimates that long-term use is unlikely to be more than 5% of the risk of smoking.[12]

Nicotine is a cause of dependence, but contrary to popular belief, it has only relatively minor harmful effects from normal use . Nicotine does not cause cancer,[13] heart[14] or lung disease.[15] These diseases are caused by smoking tobacco.

All vaporisers consist of two basic parts: a battery (usually rechargeable) and a tank or pod which holds the e-liquid (e-juice) and heating 'coil'.

Components of a vaporiser

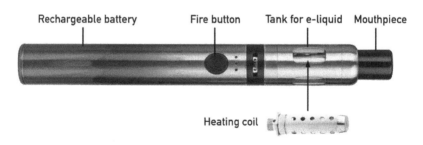

Parts of a (vape pen) vaporiser

A cotton 'wick' draws e-liquid from the tank or pod onto the coil. When you breathe in or press a button, the battery heats the coil, vaporising the e-liquid into an aerosol.

E-liquid consists of nicotine and flavourings (both optional) mixed with propylene glycol (PG) and vegetable glycerine (VG). Most users start with tobacco flavoured e-liquid. However, there are many other flavours and most switch to fruit, sweet or mint over time.[16]

Vapers typically use their device instead of having a cigarette, for example, first thing in the morning, with a cup of coffee or after a stressful event, with the aim of weaning themselves off deadly smoking products.

Vaping is unique as a quitting aid in that it delivers nicotine as well as replicating many aspects of smoking behaviour and helps you cope with smoking triggers, such as the smell of smoke or having a drink. It also may help to prevent relapse.[10]

Most former smokers who vape find it more or equally satisfying as smoking.[17] Smokers who switch to vaping are healthier, feel and smell better, are protecting the health of people around them and have a lot more money in their pockets. The typical cost of vaping in Australia is around 10% of the cost of smoking.

Vaping should not be taken up by non-smokers, especially young people who don't smoke. Vaping exposes non-smokers to an increased risk of harm to their health.

Tobacco harm reduction

Long-term quitting is a difficult task for many smokers, even with the best treatments. Most smokers cycle repeatedly through periods of quitting and relapse over many years. As a result, many continue to smoke and remain at high risk of serious illness and an early death. Currently, nearly three million Australians still smoke.[5]

Vaping is a form of 'tobacco harm reduction' (THR) for smokers who are otherwise unable or unwilling to quit.[18] THR involves replacing high-risk combustible tobacco products such as cigarettes with lower-risk, non-combustible nicotine alternatives, like vaping, heated-tobacco products or Swedish snus.

Tobacco harm reduction is based on the principle that people smoke for the effects of nicotine, while the real risks are caused by the toxic components in the smoke. The focus is on reducing harm, not on eliminating nicotine. THR also protects bystanders from second-hand smoke.

THR is not a replacement for traditional quitting strategies but is a supplementary approach to reduce harm in those who would otherwise continue to smoke.[19]

All nicotine products fall on a scale of risk (see the figure below).[20] On the right of the figure are the deadliest products which involve burning tobacco, such as cigarettes, pipes and cigars. On the left are low-risk, non-combustible nicotine products such as nicotine patches, nicotine gum and e-cigarettes. Smokers who switch to vaping can continue to enjoy nicotine and the 'smoking' ritual but with a dramatically reduced risk to their health.

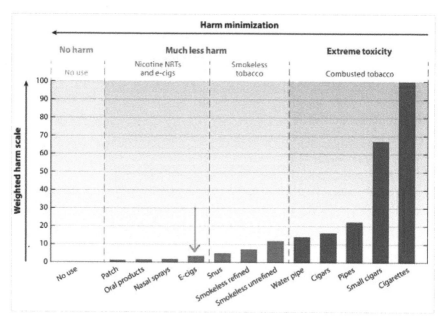

The risk continuum of nicotine products
Adapted from Nutt et al. 2014[21] and reproduced from Abrams et al. 2018[22]

Harm reduction strategies for risky behaviours are widely used in public health. We accept that some heroin users cannot quit and provide them with methadone or buprenorphine as safer (not 'safe') alternatives. Intravenous drug users are given clean needles to prevent HIV/AIDS and other infections. Motorcycle helmets reduce the risk of head injury. Car drivers and passengers are protected by seat belts and airbags. Substituting vaping nicotine for smoking to reduce harm is no different, yet it evokes powerful opposition in some circles.

The federal government has long been reluctant to spend sufficient money on smoking cessation and tobacco control. An added benefit of vaping as a quitting strategy is that it involves minimal public expenditure. All costs are paid by the user. And a flourishing vaping industry could generate employment, taxes and a huge saving to the health care system.

A legitimate quitting method

The best option for your health is always to quit smoking and nicotine altogether. However, if you can't quit with conventional treatments, vaping nicotine is an effective alternative. The Royal Australian College of General Practitioners reviewed all the evidence and recognised that there is a valid role for vaping nicotine:

> 'For people who have tried to achieve smoking cessation with first-line therapy (combination of behavioural support and TGA-approved pharmacotherapy) but failed and are still motivated to quit smoking, NVPs [Nicotine Vaping Products] may be a reasonable intervention to recommend along with behavioural support.'[4]

In 2020, the federal government acknowledged that smokers should have the choice to switch to vaping nicotine. Nicotine liquid can now be sold from Australian chemist shops and online pharmacies.[23]

Vaping nicotine is strongly supported by New Zealand, UK and Canadian health authorities. According to the New Zealand Ministry of

Health, 'Vaping has helped many people quit smoking and is a legitimate way to become smoke-free.'[24]

Vaping nicotine is also endorsed by a wide range of international medical and health organisations, including the Royal Australian and New Zealand College of Psychiatrists, the British Medical Association, the French National Academy of Medicine and the New Zealand Medical Association. See the Appendix for a list of supporting organisations.

Senator Hollie Hughes

Hollie is a federal senator and was Chair of the 2020 Senate Inquiry into Tobacco Harm Reduction. Like many smokers, she quit 'accidentally' with vaping.

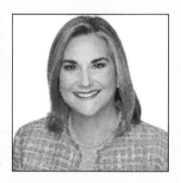

'I smoked socially for twenty years. I enjoyed the physical ritual, taking time out with a cigarette, having a glass of wine and relaxing.

In early 2020, the health minister announced that it would be basically illegal to vape in Australia. Whilst I didn't know much about vaping or how it could be used as a smoking cessation aid, I did know about personal choice and responsibility.

A number of my colleagues and I gained a reprieve on that legislation, but I also set to work on a Senate Inquiry into Tobacco Harm Reduction — essentially, vaping.

It was at this stage I met with a doctor to learn more about this whole vaping caper. He went through a thorough consultation — why and when I smoked, triggers and stressors and all that. I still had no intention to quit.

I tried several different types of vapes, flavours and strengths in the doctor's office. I left that day armed with a small pod vape, a few tobacco-flavoured pods at the weakest nicotine strength (1.8%) and a prescription.

Using pods is a more expensive way to vape, but at $8.50 per pod versus $58 for a packet of cigarettes I am still miles ahead, and for me it is clean and easy.

As I write today, I have not had a cigarette for 235 days — in fact, the thought of smoking makes me quite ill, let alone the smell. I still enjoy the social ritual, now with a pleasant tropical flavour, but without the toxic chemicals.

As an adult, you should be able to consume nicotine how you choose - gum, lozenge, spray, patch, vape — and even a cigarette. It's your choice. The ideological objection to vaping is still something I find absurd in a liberal society.

I look forward to one day being able to buy my nicotine pods from a local vape store, rather than having to order from an overseas-based business.'

http://www.holliehughes.com.au/

2

VAPING IN AUSTRALIA

Take-home messages

- Over half a million Australians now vape
- Regular vapers are almost exclusively current or former smokers
- Australia's harsh regulation of vaping is out of step with other western countries
- Australia is the only western democracy to ban the sale and use of nicotine liquid without a prescription
- It is legal to vape nicotine if you have a prescription from a registered Australian medical practitioner
- The UK and NZ governments actively promote vaping as a legitimate quitting tool

Despite harsh regulations, vaping nicotine in Australia is increasingly popular. In 2019, 2.5% of Australians or 522,000 people were vaping at least monthly.[5] This is a substantial increase from 2016 when 1.2% of Australians or 238,000 people were vaping.[25]

Australian vaping rates are low by international standards. Adult vaping rates are 5.7% of the population in Great Britain,[26] 4.7% in New Zealand[27] and 3.2% in the USA.[28] In 2020, an estimated 68 million people were vaping globally and millions of others have quit both smoking and vaping.[29]

Vaping is the most popular aid for quitting or reducing smoking in Australia. In 2019, 22% of Australian smokers used vaping to quit or cut down, 16.8% used nicotine replacement products, 10.2% asked their doctor for help and 6.3% used a smoking cessation pill.[5] Only 1.8% called the Quitline.

Vaping is most popular in young adults, the age group likely to get the most benefit from switching from smoking. In 2019, 10% of eighteen- to twenty-four-year-olds were vaping. However, vaping is used by smokers of all ages.

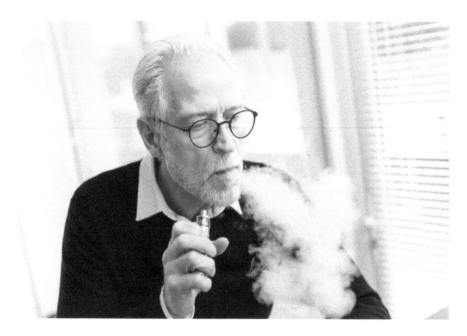

Vaping is suitable for adult smokers of all ages

Regular vaping is almost exclusively confined to current or former smokers and is rare in people who have not previously smoked. Fewer than 0.3% of Australians who had never smoked were vaping weekly or more often in 2019.[5]

The main reasons for vaping by Australian smokers are to quit (44%), to cut down (24%), to reduce harm (23%) and to prevent relapse to smoking (19%).[5]

Cost savings for Australian smokers

How much of your hard-earned money goes up in smoke each year? Australia has the highest cigarette prices in the world.[30] The price of a pack of twenty cigarettes of the leading brand is thirty-five dollars, so a pack-a-day smoker spends over $12,500 every year on smoking!

Calculate how much you spend on smoking with ATHRA's Smoking Cost Calculator here: www.athra.org.au/smoking-cost-calculator/.

The cost of vaping is about 5-25% of the cost of smoking depending on the type of vaping device and e-liquid used. This table is a guide to the annual cost savings for different vaping products compared to smoking.

Annual costs of smoking and vaping					
Smoking	Pack of 20 cigarettes $35 daily[30]			Annual cost $12,775	
Vaping	**Vaping devices**	**E-liquid**	**Accessories**	**Annual cost**	**Annual saving**
Pre-filled pod vape	Three devices, $90	Pods. 1 daily, $2,920		$3,060	$9,765
Re-fillable vape pen with premixed e-liquid	Three vape pens, $150	E-liquid, in 120 ml bottles (5ml per day), $620	Coils, replaced every 2 weeks, $100	$870	$11,905

Re-fillable vape pen with DIY e-liquid	Three vape pens, $150	E-liquid ingredients: PG, VG, nicotine, flavouring (5ml per day), $200	Coils replaced every 2 weeks, gloves, pipettes, syringes, bottles, scales, $350	$600	$12,175

What could you do with those savings? Imagine an overseas holiday each year or finally paying off the credit card bill or home mortgage? It would be like giving yourself a huge pay rise!

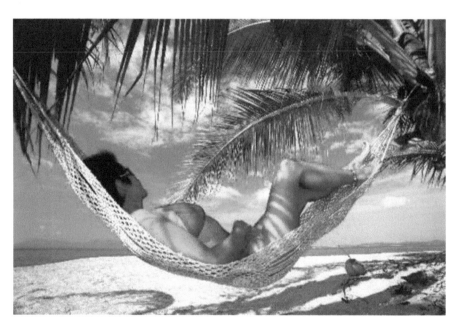

A tropical holiday every year or continuing to smoke?

Australia's policy on vaping

Australian authorities have taken a virtually prohibitionist attitude to vaping, discouraging its use, banning the sale of nicotine liquid in vape shops and requiring a doctor's prescription to vape legally. In other western countries such as New Zealand, the UK, US, European Union and Canada, nicotine liquid is a consumer product and can be purchased by adults at retail outlets without a prescription. In Australia it is easier to buy deadly tobacco cigarettes than the far safer and cheaper alternative.

The restrictive Australian laws make it very hard to access nicotine liquid legally, especially for the high-risk and vulnerable groups that need it most — those with mental illness, Indigenous people, lower socio-economic groups, people who use drugs and homeless people. This de facto prohibition has criminalised hundreds of thousands of users and created a thriving black-market for nicotine liquids.

Australian health authorities have raised concerns about the threat to young people, tobacco industry involvement, child poisoning and unknown long-term risks of vaping. Some of these concerns are legitimate and are discussed in more detail in Part 3.

The media has amplified these concerns. Alarming, catchy headlines attract more readers and advertising dollars but are often misleading. Priority is given to negative stories that exaggerate risks and often misrepresent the scientific evidence.[31] The benefits of vaping and its potential to save the lives of many thousands of adult Australian smokers is rarely mentioned.

There is a strong prohibitionist, coercive and punitive attitude to smoking in Australia. Just like the 'war on drugs', authorities have a zero-tolerance policy for tobacco, nicotine and anything that looks like smoking. Smokers should just quit smoking and nicotine and those who continue to smoke are punished with eye-watering tobacco taxes and stigmatisation. The war on smoking and the tobacco industry has become a moral crusade against vaping as well.

In opposing vaping, the Australian government is not complying with its own guidelines. Tobacco harm reduction is one of the three pillars of

Australia's National Tobacco Strategy to 'reduce harm associated with continuing use of tobacco and nicotine products'.[32]

Australia is also obligated to support tobacco harm reduction as a signatory to the World Health Organisation's Framework Convention on Tobacco Control (FCTC).[33] The FCTC requires Australia to not only allow reduced-risk products but actively promote them.[33] In the introduction, article 1(d) of the FCTC defines tobacco control as:

> 'a range of supply, demand and harm reduction strategies that aim to improve the health of a population by eliminating or reducing their consumption of tobacco products and exposure to tobacco smoke.'[33]

The hostility of the health minister, Greg Hunt, to vaping has been clear since his famous comment in September 2019, 'The most important thing I do as health minister is not to allow this nicotine into Australia'.[34]

It is not known why the health minister has formed this view. However, his persistent opposition has been the main driver of government policy, despite considerable support for vaping by his colleagues in the Liberal and National coalition.

It is no wonder that most Australians are misinformed about vaping.[35] If the government and most health and medical organisations repeatedly oppose vaping, why wouldn't you believe them? Their mission is to improve public health. It is natural to assume that they are following the evidence and have our best interests at heart.

Unfortunately, Australia's policy on vaping is driven less by the scientific evidence and more by ideological, political and moral arguments. This is discussed in more detail in Part 3.

Is nicotine e-liquid legal in Australia?

Possessing nicotine

It is legal to possess or use nicotine e-liquid in Australia if you have a prescription from a registered Australian medical practitioner.

Purchasing nicotine

Nicotine e-liquid can be legally accessed in two ways with a doctor's prescription.

Personal Importation Scheme

Nicotine liquid can be purchased from international websites and imported into Australia for personal use under the Therapeutic Goods Administration (TGA) Personal Importation Scheme.[36] You can order up to three months' supply at a time to help you quit or reduce smoking, up to a total of fifteen months' supply each year.

Australian pharmacies

Nicotine can be purchased from participating Australian chemist shops and online pharmacies.[37] This requires a prescription from a doctor who is an Authorised Prescriber for nicotine.[38]

Nicotine liquid cannot be legally sold by other retail outlets such as vape shops or tobacconists.

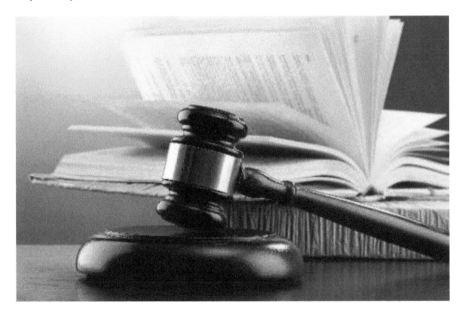

It is illegal to possess liquid nicotine unless it is prescribed by a doctor

Penalties

Possessing or using nicotine liquid without a prescription is a criminal offence in all states and territories and is punishable by steep fines and potential prison terms.

State	Penalty	Prison term	Legislation
ACT	$32,000 max or prison or both	2 years	Medicines, Poisons and Therapeutic Goods Act 2008, 4.1.3, 36
Western Australia	$30,000		Medicines and Poisons Act 2014, 2.16.2 and 115
Victoria	$1,817		Drugs, Poisons and Controlled Substances Regulations 1981, 36B
South Australia	$10,000 max		Controlled Substances Act 1984, 4.22
Northern Territory	$15,700 max or prison	12 months	Medicines, Poisons and Therapeutic Goods Act, 2.2, Div 3, 44.2
Queensland	$27,570 max		Medicines and Poisons Act 2019, 2.1.1.34
New South Wales	$2,200 max or prison or both	6 months	Poisons and Therapeutic Goods Act 1966, No 31, 16
Tasmania	$8,650 or prison	Up to 2 years	Poisons Act 1971, Part 3, Division 1, Clause 36

Penalties for nicotine possession

State and territory laws

The states and territories regulate the sale of vaping products, vaping in public places and cars, and the minimum age of purchase. Ironically, vaping products are regulated more strictly than tobacco products although they are substantially less harmful. Regulations are a little different between states and territories, but in general, the following rules apply across Australia:[39]

- Vaping is not allowed in smoke-free areas
- The sale of nicotine liquid is illegal, except from a pharmacy with a prescription
- The sale of nicotine-free e-liquid to adults is legal but is not permitted under the age of eighteen years
- The display of vaping products in a vape shop is banned in most states
- The sale of vaporisers to adults is legal except in Western Australia where the sale of vaping devices which resemble tobacco products is banned
- It is an offence to sell vaping products and accessories to minors (under eighteen years)
- It is also an offence for adults to purchase products for a minor
- Vaping is banned in cars with children under the age of sixteen years
- Internet sales are banned in South Australia
- It is legal for adults to possess or use a vaporiser without nicotine

Comparison to similar countries

New Zealand and the United Kingdom have similar tobacco control policies and smoking rates to Australia but have come to starkly different positions on vaping nicotine. Both countries actively encourage smokers to switch to vaping nicotine.

New Zealand

On 10 August 2021, the New Zealand Parliament passed legislation to legalise and regulate nicotine vaping.[40] Nicotine e-liquid is available as an adult consumer product from vape shops and general retail stores. The Associate Health Minister Dr Ayesha Verrall said at the time:

'It strikes a balance between ensuring these products are not marketed or sold to young people, while ensuring vaping products are available for smokers who want to switch to a less harmful alternative.'[41]

The New Zealand Ministry of Health encourages stop-smoking services and health workers to support smokers in switching to vaping.[42]

In 2021, the New Zealand government launched the Vape to Quit Strong campaign to promote vaping.[43] The campaign features television and radio promotions in prime time, posters and social media banners.

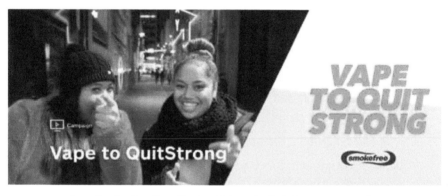

A poster for the New Zealand Vape to Quit Strong campaign

The Ministry of Health has also established a website, *Vaping Facts* at www.vapingfacts.health.nz to help smokers make an informed choice about whether to vape or not.[24]

There is widespread support for vaping in New Zealand from government and leading health and medical organisations (Appendix).

United Kingdom

Vaping nicotine is an integral part of tobacco control policy in the United Kingdom, with strong support from Parliament,[44] the National Health Service[45] and Public Health England,[46] the government's public health agency. Vaping is also a key part of Stoptober, Public Health England's stop-smoking campaign held each year in October.[47]

According to Public Health England, 'nicotine vaping products could play a crucial role in reducing the enormous health burden caused by cigarette smoking.'[46]

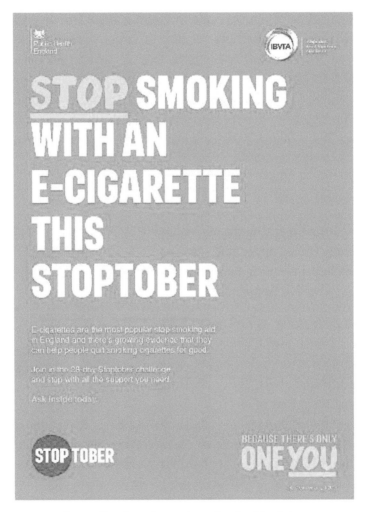

Promotion for using e-cigarettes for Stoptober
This image is subject to crown copyright. On clarification of interpretation of the regulations, the Committees on Advertising and Practice (CAP) in the UK deemed that joint campaigns between trade bodies and public health stakeholders were not legal.

Vaping is endorsed by almost all health and medical organisations in the UK, such as the British Medical Association, British Lung Foundation, British Heart Foundation, the Royal College of General Practitioners and the Royal Society for Public Health. See the Appendix for a full list.

Vaping is by far the most popular quitting aid in the UK and is used in one in three quit attempts.[6] Vaping is largely confined to current and former smokers and 'e-cigarette use by never smokers remains negligible'.[6]

The decline in smoking rates in the UK has accelerated since vaping became popular, as more smokers make the transition to the safer alternative.[26]

Joe Hildebrand

Joe is a journalist and media personality who 'knew I could never quit' smoking. He switched to vaping five years ago and has never felt better.

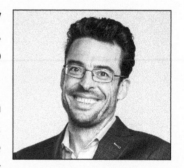

'I started smoking when I was fifteen and a massive nerd trying to be cool. It was the stupidest thing I have ever done and there is some strong competition in that field.

For the next twenty-five years smoking was a part of me. Every cigarette was like an extension of my fingers. What non-smokers often don't understand is that smoking isn't just an addiction. It's something that's built into everything else you do in life.

I would smoke with my morning coffee and my evening beer. I would smoke to celebrate getting together with a girl and to commiserate breaking up with her. I would smoke while waiting for the train, bus and taxi. I would smoke while writing, reading and watching. Smoking wasn't just an accessory to those things; it was a part of them.

I knew I could never quit and so I tried to cut down to only those cigarettes I couldn't live without. Ultimately these were ones that went with beer.

It was at a work function that I realised even this was not enough as I huddled alone down the bottom of the garden. A girl at the party noticed this and handed me a small cylindrical vape. It looked, felt and acted like a cigarette. It filled the empty space where the cigarette used to be.

A few weeks later I stubbed out my last cigarette. That was five years ago.

These days that vape is still where my cigarette used to be. I use it only in the evenings when I am having a drink. I no longer cough and hack. My lungs no longer burn when I run, and I run every day. I feel healthier and fitter than I did decades ago.

Almost all of my friends used to smoke. Almost all of them now vape instead. And whenever I'm talking to a smoker who's looking a bit forlorn, I tell them the exact same thing the girl at the party told me.

'Try this,' she said. 'It's a cigarette that doesn't kill you.' That was five years ago.'

3

BUSTING THE MYTHS ABOUT NICOTINE

Take-home messages

- Nicotine is a toxic poison in a highly concentrated form, however the low concentrations used in smoking and vaping cause little harm
- Almost all the harm from smoking is caused by the 7,000 toxic chemicals in smoke released from burning tobacco
- Nicotine does NOT cause cancer, lung disease or heart disease
- Dependence on nicotine is strongest when smoked, but is much less when taken in other ways such as vaping and even less in nicotine replacement therapy
- There is no evidence so far that nicotine is harmful in human adolescents or pregnant women
- Nicotine improves concentration, memory and alertness, reduces stress and helps control weight
- Nicotine can be beneficial for people with schizophrenia, Parkinson's disease, ulcerative colitis and attention deficit hyperactivity disorder (ADHD)

Nicotine has an image problem. It is the most well-known chemical in tobacco smoke and many people incorrectly believe it is the main cause of the death and illness from smoking as well. Even doctors are confused. In a recent US study, most doctors 'strongly agreed' that nicotine directly contributes to the development of cardiovascular disease (83%), COPD-emphysema (81%), and cancer (80.5%).[48]

Nicotine is habit-forming but is otherwise relatively benign and has some positive effects. Let's find out more and bust some myths!

What is nicotine?

Nicotine is a chemical found in the leaf of the tobacco plant and in smaller amounts in eggplant, tomato, potato and capsicum. Nicotine is a natural insecticide, protecting plants from various insects and other pests. It has also been used as a commercial insecticide in the past, but many insects have now developed resistance to it.

Nicotine has been used for its rewarding effects for thousands of years. The first evidence of cultivation of the tobacco plant was perhaps 6-8,000 years ago in South America.[49] In Australia, Indigenous people in Central Australia have traditionally chewed wild tobacco plants for the effects of nicotine.[50] 'Pituri' is made by Indigenous Australians by breaking up tobacco leaves into pieces, mixing with ash and chewing to form a 'quid' which is held in the mouth or cheek pocket for extended periods.

When a cigarette is smoked, nicotine is rapidly carried in the bloodstream to the brain where it releases the 'pleasure hormone' dopamine, creating the 'nicotine hit' you enjoy with the first cigarette of the day.[51] With repeated doses of nicotine, the brain becomes accustomed to the effects of nicotine and you crave further hits. Within a few hours of the last cigarette, you experience nicotine withdrawal symptoms such as irritability, anger and difficulty concentrating and sleeping, which can be relieved by smoking another cigarette. And so, the cycle continues...

Nicotine dependence or addiction?

This book refers to vaping nicotine as a 'dependence' and tobacco smoking as an 'addiction'. This difference may seem petty but is actually very important. According to the US National Institute on Drug Abuse:[52]

- Dependence means that when you stop using a drug, you experience physical 'withdrawal' symptoms. Stopping nicotine can cause anxiety, irritability and difficulty concentrating. Similarly, coffee drinkers may experience headaches, tiredness, difficulty concentrating and nausea when they reduce their caffeine intake.

- Addiction is much more serious. If you are addicted to a drug, you lose control of your drug taking and are compelled to use it, **despite knowing that it is having harmful effects**. Tobacco smoking is a true addiction as the majority of smokers know it is very dangerous, often try unsuccessfully to quit and keep smoking.

As we shall see, nicotine itself has minor effects at low doses and vaping nicotine is a relatively low-risk behaviour. You may be dependent on nicotine or vaping, but you are not addicted to it.

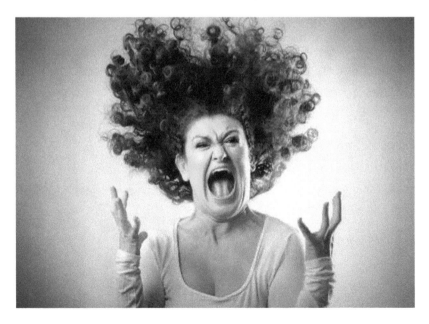

'Nicotine withdrawal is an unpleasant experience!'

Is nicotine harmful to the body?

Nicotine is a toxic poison in its highly concentrated form but the low concentrations in smoke and vapour cause little harm with normal use.

Almost all the harm from smoking is caused by over 7,000 toxic chemicals in the smoke released from burning tobacco, not by the nicotine.[11] In 1976, pioneering tobacco researcher Dr Michael Russell wrote in the *British Medical Journal*, 'people smoke for nicotine but die from the tar.' [53]

This is still thought to be true today and is supported by leading health organisations, however it is possible that harmful effects may be identified in the future.

Statements from leading health organisations

UK Royal College of Physicians[12]

'Use of nicotine alone, in the doses used by smokers, represents little if any hazard to the user.'

UK Royal Society for Public Health[54]

'Tobacco contains nicotine along with many other chemicals, but nicotine by itself is fairly harmless.'

Public Health England[55]

'Nicotine use per se represents minimal risk of serious harm to physical health and ... its addictiveness depends on how it is administered.'

New Zealand Ministry of Health[24]

'For people who smoke:
- nicotine itself is low harm
- nicotine has little or no long-term health effects

- nicotine is addictive and if your vape contains nicotine you will still be addicted to this
- it's what comes with the nicotine that could be harmful.'

National Health Service, UK[45]

'While nicotine is the addictive substance in cigarettes, it is relatively harmless.'

Nicotine does not cause cancer or lung disease and plays only a minor role in heart disease.

Cancer from smoking is caused by over seventy known cancer-causing chemicals in tobacco smoke, not nicotine.[13] Nicotine does not cause cancer in humans according to leading health authorities including the World Health Organisation's International Agency for Research on Cancer,[13] the UK Royal College of Physicians [12] and the US Surgeon General.[15]

Nicotine is also not the main cause of heart disease from smoking. Nicotine increases the heart rate and blood pressure and narrows the blood vessels, much like mild exercise. Nicotine may exacerbate existing heart conditions and can trigger an irregular heartbeat in some cases. However, the effects are minor compared to tobacco smoking.[14] Australian guidelines advise that 'All forms of nicotine replacement therapy can be used safely in stable cardiovascular disease.'[4]

There is also no evidence that nicotine itself causes lung damage or disease.[15]

Nicotine replacement therapy (patches, gum, lozenges, spray and inhalator) is generally regarded as safe. It is approved for use in Australia from the age of twelve as well as in pregnancy and is freely available from supermarkets and petrol stations. Serious side effects are rare.[56]

Nicotine reduces the blood flow to wounds and can delay healing, for example after surgery. However, studies in surgical patients have found that patients using nicotine replacement medication have better healing than those who continue to smoke.[57]

Nicotine can raise blood glucose levels and could increase the risk of diabetes.

Nicotine can be absorbed through the skin, but the concentrations used in vaping liquids are very unlikely to cause harm even after significant skin exposure.[58]

Is long-term use of nicotine harmful?

We know that the long-term use of nicotine is low-risk from decades of use of 'Swedish snus'. Snus is a moist, pasteurised, finely-ground form of tobacco usually sold in a pouch like a small teabag. It is placed under the upper lip where it slowly releases similar levels of nicotine to tobacco smoking.

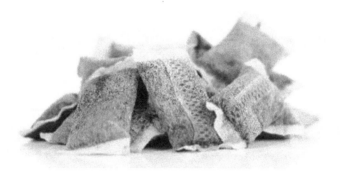

Swedish snus - small pouches of moist tobacco

Snus is used widely in Sweden as a safer alternative to smoking, however it is banned in other European countries. It is the most popular and most effective quitting aid used by men in Sweden and it is often continued long-term.[59]

There is no evidence that the long-term use of snus causes cancer, lung or heart disease. A review by Public Health England concluded that 'long-term use of nicotine as snus ... has not been found to increase the risk of serious health problems in adults.'[55]

Swedish men have the lowest smoking rate in Europe and by far the lowest rate of death from smoking in Europe.[60]

There is also no evidence of harm from long-term use of nicotine in nicotine replacement therapy. According to the Australian RACGP smoking cessation guidelines, 'Current scientific evidence does not support an association between long-term NRT (nicotine replacement therapy) exposure and serious adverse health effects.'[4]

How strong is dependence on nicotine?

Dependence on nicotine varies with how it is administered, how quickly it reaches the brain and how much is used.[61]

Nicotine is most potent from smoking because high doses get to the brain very quickly, within ten to fifteen seconds — faster than intravenously injected heroin.

Vaping and nicotine replacement therapy deliver nicotine more slowly and usually to lower levels. Many studies have found that vaping nicotine causes less dependence than smoking.[62] Nicotine gum and patches also have a very low risk of dependence.[63]

Why not just use nicotine replacement therapy?

The quit rates from nicotine replacement therapy (NRT) are very modest indeed, and most smokers have tried them repeatedly without success. In clinical trials, using a single product such as a nicotine patch has a quit rate of 6% after six to twelve months.[64] Combining two products (such as the nicotine patch and gum) increases the quit rate to 11%.[64] Nicotine products purchased over-the-counter without counselling and support are even less effective.[4]

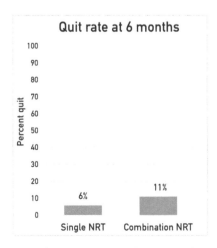

Quit rates from nicotine replacement therapy[64]

NRT provides too little nicotine too slowly for most users and often does not satisfy cravings. Most people also stop NRT too soon after quitting smoking[65] and NRT has been criticised for its inability to prevent relapse.[66] Fifty per cent of smokers who make it to six months will relapse eventually.

According to Professor Jed Rose from Duke University, who invented the nicotine patch, 'nicotine is not enough' to break tobacco addiction for many people.[70, 71] The hand-to-mouth habit, smoking triggers and the sensations of smoking (taste and 'throat hit') play a critical role in maintaining the addiction.

Vaping mimics the smoking ritual and sensations and can help to cope with smoking triggers, such as having coffee or when socialising. It can also deliver nicotine more rapidly and in higher doses than NRT. Because it is more enjoyable than NRT it is likely to be used for longer.

Is nicotine harmful in pregnancy?

Nicotine has been linked to harmful effects on the foetus in mouse and rat studies. However, there is no clear evidence that these findings apply to humans.[67]

Nicotine replacement products such as patches, gums and lozenges are approved for use in pregnancy in Australia and have been used for decades. Human studies have not shown any clear harms such as stillbirth, premature birth, low birthweight, admissions to neonatal intensive care, caesarean section, congenital abnormalities or neonatal death.[68, 69]

Nicotine may not be completely safe for the pregnant mother and foetus, but it is always safer than smoking.[70]

Positive effects of nicotine

Many smokers enjoy the effects of nicotine.[71] Nicotine releases the pleasure hormone 'dopamine' in the brain creating pleasure and a sense of reward. It also releases other brain chemicals which have positive effects.[57]

You may have noticed that nicotine improves your concentration, alertness and memory.[72] It also has a temporary calming effect and can improve your mood.[73]

Nicotine reduces your appetite and can help to reduce weight gain. When smokers quit, they put on three kilograms on average over a five-year period, although some gain a lot more.[74] Smokers who switch to vaping frequently put on less weight because they continue to use nicotine.[75]

Nicotine can improve attention and memory for people with schizophrenia.[76] Nicotine also reduces the sleepiness and weight gain caused by many of the medicines used for schizophrenia.

Nicotine improves mental performance and behaviour in some people with attention deficit hyperactivity disorder (ADHD).[77] People with ADHD often report that their condition gets worse when they stop nicotine.[78]

In people living with Parkinson's disease, nicotine may protect the brain cells from deterioration and can improve mood, attention, movement and memory.[79] Smokers are significantly less likely to get Parkinson's disease, possibly because of nicotine.[80] Nicotine may also slow the decline in mental function in Alzheimer's disease.[79]

Smokers are less likely to get ulcerative colitis, a serious inflammation of the bowel.[81] If they do get the disease, it is usually milder. It is likely that nicotine is a protective factor.

Nicotine also increases the pain threshold and reduces pain. This may be of benefit to people with chronic painful conditions.[82]

Robert Richter QC

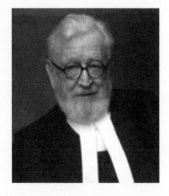

Robert is a 75-year-old criminal barrister from Melbourne, known as the 'Red Baron'.

He smoked a pack of cigarettes a day for fifty-five years, desperately trying and failing to quit on numerous occasions.

'I have been through many attempts at abstinence, hypnosis, psychotherapy, patches, lozenges, nicotine gum. I simply found that smoking, for me, was indispensable in allowing me to concentrate on work and to sleep. Without nicotine I could not run my legal practice.'

Three years ago, Robert was diagnosed with a very nasty form of lung cancer. Fortunately, the tumour was very small and was surgically removed. The surgeon told him never to smoke again. When Robert asked about vaping, he was told it would not damage his lungs and that 'it was ninety-five per cent safer than smoking cigarettes.'

'I switched to vaping then and there and have not had a cigarette since.'

Vaping helped him quit, gave him the nicotine he needed and was not offensive to others. He says it was a no-brainer.

'I have no intention to quit vaping as I would also have to retire from practice as a barrister and I don't want to retire,' he told me. 'I need the nicotine to function, and the patches or gum just don't cut it.'

Robert's objective was to find the most efficient vaporiser and e-liquid which produced the least vapour cloud and lasts all day. He uses a mint flavoured e-liquid in a compact re-fillable pod vape which does all that.

'My message for other smoker addicts is to try vaping nicotine if they have been unable to quit with other methods. It is the only thing that I found acceptable and allowed me to function normally. Be sure to buy from a safe and reliable supplier.'

He also cautions non-smokers that vaping is not for them: 'If you are not a nicotine addict already or a vaper of any kind, don't start.'

4

IS VAPING SAFER THAN SMOKING?

Take-home messages

- Vaping nicotine is not harmless, but there is overwhelming scientific agreement that it is far less harmful than smoking
- Smokers who switch to vaping are exposed to far fewer toxins
- The cancer risk from vaping is less than one two hundredth of the risk from smoking
- There is no evidence that vaping causes heart disease
- Smokers who switch to vaping have improved lung health
- Vaping does not cause 'popcorn lung'
- The outbreak of deaths and serious lung disease in the US called EVALI was caused by vaping contaminated illicit cannabis oils, not nicotine vaping products
- There is no evidence so far that vaping is harmful to bystanders
- The long-term risk of vaping is unlikely to be more than 5% of the risk of smoking
- Vaping is almost certain to be safer than smoking in pregnancy
- Vaping nicotine is less likely to cause dependence than smoking
- Accidental swallowing of nicotine by children is rare, and most cases result in little harm
- Fires and explosions from lithium-ion batteries are rare and most can be prevented

Most people incorrectly believe that vaping is as harmful as or more harmful than smoking. Vaping looks like smoking and it is easy to assume that it also causes serious harm. Misinformation by vaping sceptics and alarmist media coverage reinforce that belief.

However, there is overwhelming scientific evidence that vaping nicotine is far less harmful than smoking tobacco. Cigarette smoke is a poisonous mix of over 7,000 chemicals caused by burning tobacco at temperatures up to 900°C.[11] It is these toxins, including carbon monoxide and over seventy carcinogens, carried in solid smoke and tar particles and hot gases, which cause almost all the harm from smoking.

In contrast, vaping involves heating a liquid solution to about 250°C into tiny liquid droplets, without tobacco, combustion or smoke. Vapour has been shown to contain propylene glycol, vegetable glycerine, oxidants, volatile organic compounds, some metals, nicotine, flavour chemicals and minimal or no carbon monoxide.[83] However, the vast majority of toxic chemicals and solid particles in smoke are not found in vapour.

A comprehensive review by Public Health England concluded that the concentrations of toxins in vapour are mostly below 1% of those in smoke and far below the levels which are known to cause harm to the body and that 'on current evidence, there is no doubt that smokers who switch to vaping reduce the risks to their health dramatically.' [84]

The peak US scientific body, the National Academies of Sciences, Engineering and Medicine (NASEM) also concluded that 'there is conclusive evidence that completely substituting NVPs (nicotine vaping products) for combustible tobacco cigarettes reduces users' exposure to numerous toxicants and carcinogens present in combustible tobacco cigarettes.'[85]

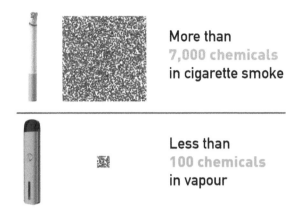

More than

7,000 chemicals

in cigarette smoke

Less than

100 chemicals

in vapour

Comparing the number of chemicals in smoke vs vapour

Comparing vaping nicotine to smoking

Asking if vaping is safe is the wrong question. Nothing is completely safe. Every product we use has some risk and adults are constantly making risk-benefit decisions before using medicines and/or other products.

As vaping nicotine is almost exclusively used by smokers, any risk should be compared to the risk of continuing to smoke. Comprehensive reviews by leading, independent health organisations agree that vaping is considerably less harmful than smoking.

Country	Organisation	Risk from vaping
UK	UK Royal College of Physicians, 2016[12]	Vaping is at least 95% less risky than smoking
	Public Health England, 2018[55]	
	The UK Committee on Toxicity of Chemicals in Food, Consumer Products, and the Environment (COT), 2020[86]	Vaping is 'significantly less harmful than combustible tobacco cigarettes'

US	National Academies of Sciences, Engineering and Medicine, 2018[85]	Vaping is 'likely to be far less harmful' than smoking.
New Zealand	The New Zealand Ministry of Health, 2020[24]	Vaping is 'not harmless, but it is much less harmful than smoking'
Canada	Centre for Addiction and Mental Health, Canada 2021[87]	'Switching completely to e-cigarettes will significantly reduce the harms associated with combusted tobacco'
	Health Canada, 2020[88]	'Vaping is less harmful than smoking'

The UK Royal College of Physicians stated in more detail:

'Although it is not possible to precisely quantify the long-term health risks associated with e-cigarettes, the available data suggest that they are unlikely to exceed 5% of those associated with smoked tobacco products and may well be substantially lower than this figure.'[12]

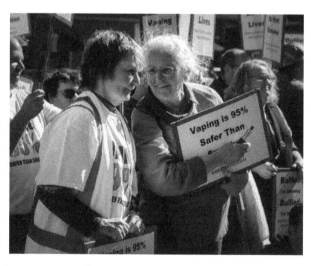

Vaping advocates at a rally in Melbourne: 'Vaping is 95% safer than smoking'

Some anti-vaping advocates contest the accuracy of this estimate without suggesting an alternative figure.[89] However, the exact figure is not the issue. The purpose of the '95% safer' estimate is to help communicate a ballpark for the level of risk so smokers can make an informed choice. Just saying vaping is 'less harmful' is too vague. That could be 30%, 60%, or maybe even 99% less harmful.

The '95% safer' estimate is based on the following scientific evidence:

1. Most of the harmful toxins in smoke are completely absent from vapour. Those that are present are at much lower concentrations.[84] If the toxins are greatly reduced, the health risks will be much lower.

2. When smokers switch to vaping, levels of toxins and carcinogens measured in the blood, saliva and urine ('biomarkers') are substantially lower and, for many toxins, are the same as in a non-smoker.[90]

3. There are substantial health improvements in smokers who switch to vaping. Risk of a heart attack reduces,[91] blood pressure falls,[92] asthma[93] and symptoms of COPD (emphysema)[94] improve and vapers typically say they just feel a lot better.

4. After 15 years of vaping nicotine in dozens of countries, there has not been one confirmed death directly caused by vaping nicotine. Serious health effects are extremely rare.

It is important to note that the risk may vary with different devices. High wattage devices expose users to more toxins and are likely to be more harmful than low powered devices.[95]

No serious authority suggests that vaping is completely harmless. Non-smokers and young people under eighteen years should not vape. However, the benefit for adult smokers is beyond reasonable doubt — if you are a smoker who cannot quit, switching to vaping nicotine will dramatically reduce your exposure to toxic chemicals and reduce the harm to your health.

Does vaping cause cancer?

Switching from smoking to vaping dramatically reduces your risk of cancer. The cancer risk from vaping nicotine has been estimated to be more than two hundred times less than the cancer risk from smoking.[96]

The carcinogens in tobacco smoke are either absent from vapour or are present at very low levels.[97] There is also a dramatic reduction of carcinogens in the blood, saliva and urine of vapers (biomarkers) compared to smokers.[98]

Studies comparing vapour to cigarette smoke have found that it is far less likely to cause damage to the genes which lead to cancer.[99]

The lung cancer risk from vaping has been estimated in one study to be 50,000 times less than from traditional cigarette smoking.[100]

According to the New Zealand Ministry of Health, 'The current estimate is, if vaping is found to be associated with cancer, the risk will only be a tiny fraction of the risks of smoking.'[24] However, the exact size of the reduction in cancer risk will only become clear after several further decades of use.

Does vaping cause heart disease?

There is no evidence that vaping causes heart disease.[14, 85] In fact, there is growing evidence that the risk of heart disease is reduced when smokers switch to vaping.[91]

Leading researchers reviewed the evidence and concluded:

'If e-cigarettes can be substituted completely for conventional cigarettes, the harms from smoking would be substantially reduced and there would likely be a substantial net benefit for cardiovascular health.'[101]

Nicotine itself has some temporary effects on the cardiovascular system, such as an increase in heart rate and blood pressure and constriction of the arteries. However, nicotine does not appear to significantly contribute to cardiovascular disease.[102, 103]

Laboratory and animal studies have shown potentially harmful effects from nicotine e-liquid and vapour.[104] However, the effects are less than from tobacco smoking and their relevance for human health remains uncertain.[105]

A widely publicised study published in 2019 claimed to show that vaping increased the risk of having a heart attack. However, this study was seriously flawed and was subsequently retracted by the journal.[106]

Does vaping cause lung disease?

Some studies have found that vaping by non-smokers may worsen asthma, bronchitis and cough.[107] In contrast, adult smokers who switch to vaping show improvements in lung symptoms,[108] breathing,[109] asthma[110] and COPD (emphysema)[94] and report fewer respiratory infections.[111]

There is no evidence that nicotine itself harms the lungs in adult smokers[15] or that it increases the risk of Covid-19.[112]

Potentially harmful effects of vaping have been found in cells in laboratory and animal studies, although these changes are far less than from smoking.[117] However, it is unclear if these findings also apply to humans. Laboratory tests often use unrealistic doses in an artificial setting and animals often respond differently to humans. As one review concluded, 'when one empirically analyses animal models using scientific tools, they fall far short of being able to predict human responses.'[113]

A widely quoted study reported that vaping caused lung disease.[114] However re-evaluation of this study confirmed that any lung harm found was caused by prior smoking and there was no evidence of harm to the lungs from vaping itself.[115]

Does vaping cause 'popcorn lung'?

Popcorn lung (bronchiolitis obliterans) is a rare, but serious lung disease first detected in popcorn factory workers exposed to high levels of 'diacetyl', used to give a buttery flavour.

Diacetyl has also been used in the past in vaping e-liquids. However, there has not been a single case of popcorn lung linked to vaping.[116] Cigarette smoke contains diacetyl at levels hundreds of times higher than vaping aerosols and there has never even been a case of the condition due to smoking.[117] Diacetyl is now rarely used and is banned in products used in Australia.[118]

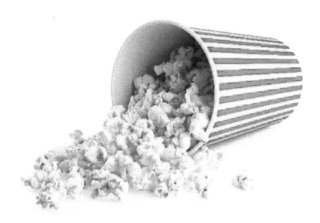

Popcorn lung?

What about the lung injury deaths in the United States?

In 2019, there was an outbreak of a serious and fatal lung condition in the United States caused by an ingredient added to black market cannabis vaping oils. This condition was known as EVALI (Electronic-cigarette or Vaping product use-Associated Lung Injury).

In early 2019, illicit cannabis suppliers started adding vitamin E acetate to dilute cannabis oils to make them go further and to increase profits. Analyses of the vaping products used and lung tissue samples detected cannabis and vitamin E acetate in almost all cases.[119] The Centres for Disease Control and Prevention (CDC) in the US identified vitamin E acetate as the primary cause of EVALI.[120] A number of people were subsequently arrested for manufacturing the illicit cannabis vapes.[121]

Not a single case of EVALI has been linked to commercial nicotine vaping products. A more appropriate name for the condition is CVALI (Cannabis Vaping Associated Lung Injury).

Does vaping cause seizures?

A small number of seizures have been reported in people who vape nicotine, but there is no evidence that vaping was the cause. Even cigarette smoking does not cause seizures. Leading researcher Professor

Neal Benowitz reviewed the evidence and concluded that it was highly unlikely that there was an increased risk of seizures from vaping.[363]

Is vaping harmful to bystanders?

Unlike second-hand smoke, there is no evidence so far that vaping is harmful to bystanders. According to Public Health England's review in 2018, 'to date there have been no identified health risks of passive vaping to bystanders.'[55] The report of the UK Royal College of Physicians in 2016 stated 'There is, so far, no direct evidence that such passive exposure is likely to cause significant harm.'[12]

Unlike smoking, the person vaping retains over 90% of the inhaled aerosol and only a very small amount of vapour is released into the surrounding air.[122] There is also no 'side-stream' vapour. Side-stream smoke (from the burning tip) accounts for at least 80% of second-hand smoke from a cigarette.

Furthermore, the liquid aerosol droplets from vapour evaporate and disperse in seconds, much more quickly than the solid particles in smoke, further reducing risk.[123]

Based on the carcinogens present and their estimated doses in second-hand vapour, the cancer risk from passive vaping was estimated to be fifty thousand times less than for passive smoking.[124]

What about unknown long-term side-effects?

Like all new products, the precise long-term health effects of vaping nicotine will not be known for another twenty or thirty years. Although we don't know everything about vaping, we already know there are far fewer toxic chemicals at much lower doses in vapour compared to smoking, there are much lower levels of toxins in the bodies of vapers, and smokers who switch to vaping nicotine show substantial health improvements.

According to the UK Royal College of Physicians, the long-term risk of vaping is unlikely to be more than 5% of the risk of smoking.[12]

Modelling studies of the future risks and benefits of vaping have predicted that vaping will have an overall positive benefit to population health. This is because the benefits of quitting by adult smokers far out-weigh any potential harms, such as their use by youth.[125]

As with any new product, it is possible that some harms may emerge over time. Continued monitoring is needed to detect any problems that may arise.

Is vaping safe in pregnancy?

There is currently little evidence on the safety of vaping in pregnancy. However, it is almost certain to be safer than smoking.

Vaping in pregnancy is endorsed by an important expert group in the UK, the Smoking in Pregnancy Challenge Group, a partnership between the Royal College of Midwives, the Royal College of Obstetricians and Gynaecologists and the Royal College of Paediatrics and Child Health.

The Challenge Group provides the following advice to midwives:

'Very little research exists regarding the safety of using e-cigarettes (vaping) during pregnancy, however evidence from adult smokers in general suggests that they are likely to be significantly less harm-ful to a pregnant woman and her baby than continuing to smoke.'[27]

The UK Royal College of Midwives 2019 Position Statement on quit-ting in pregnancy states:

'E-cigarettes contain some toxins, but at far lower levels than found in tobacco smoke. If a pregnant woman who has been smoking chooses to use an e-cigarette (vaping) and it helps her to quit smoking and stay smoke-free, she should be supported to do so.'[126]

Although it is not risk-free, vaping may have a role as a substitute for pregnant women who are otherwise unable to quit smoking. It should not be used by pregnant women who do not smoke.

Some studies of Swedish snus (small tobacco pouches held in the mouth) in pregnancy have found an increased risk of preterm delivery and preeclampsia (high blood pressure).[127] Preeclampsia is possibly linked to nicotine.

Can you become dependent on vaping?

Most vapers are already dependent on nicotine from past smoking and have transferred their nicotine dependence to a much safer product. Smokers who switch to vaping become less dependent and find it easier to quit vaping when they are ready to try.[62]

Tobacco smoking is particularly addictive because it delivers high levels of nicotine very rapidly to the brain. Vaping releases nicotine more slowly and generally at lower levels, although some modern vaping devices can deliver nicotine at a similar speed and dose to smoking.[128]

Smoke also contains other chemicals that make nicotine more addictive, for example monoamine oxidase inhibitors.[129] These chemicals are not present in vapour.

Non-smokers who start vaping nicotine can become dependent on nicotine, although this is rare in young people. For example, in a large study in the US, fewer than 4% of young never-smokers who vaped reported symptoms of dependence on vaping.[130]

How common is child poisoning?

Accidental poisoning from nicotine e-liquid is rare especially when compared to poisoning from other chemicals and medicines. Ingestion of nicotine is usually followed by intense vomiting and most cases result in little harm.

The Australian Poisons Information Centres reported on exposure to nicotine e-liquid.[131] There were 202 cases over seven years from 2009-2016, of which 36% were children. Most patients had mild symptoms with only twelve having moderate symptoms, usually gastrointestinal. There were no cases with serious side-effects and no deaths.

The Victorian Poisons Information Centre reported low rates of exposure to liquid nicotine in 2018 and 2019.[132] The number of cases referred for treatment was fourteen in 2018 and fifteen in 2019.

According to a review by Public Health England, the risk from ingestion of e-liquids appears comparable to similar potentially toxic household substances.[84]

There have been four deaths in children from nicotine poisoning reported globally in the last fifteen years. These are four deaths too many but should be compared to over 100 million people who have died from smoking-related disease during this time.

One of these deaths occurred in Australia.[133] In May 2018, an eighteen-month old child died after drinking from an open (non-childproof) bottle of concentrated nicotine (100mg/mL) when the mother was mixing the nicotine with other ingredients. This tragic case underlines the importance of allowing low-concentrations of premixed nicotine liquid to be sold in Australia, in child-resistant containers with warning labels. This would make the importation of concentrated and more toxic solutions unnecessary.

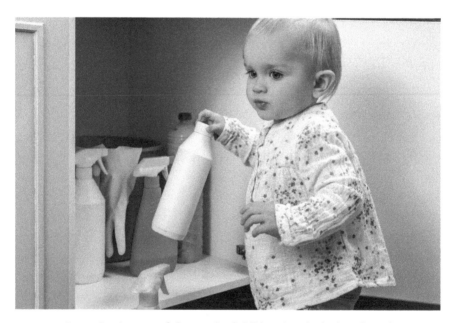

Keep nicotine out of the reach of children in a locked cupboard

Accidental nicotine poisoning of children is rare in other western countries such as the United States,[134] the United Kingdom[135] and Canada.[136] Most cases are mild and recover without treatment.

What is the risk of adult poisoning?

Adult deaths from deliberately overdosing with liquid nicotine have occurred but are very rare. Most cases result in prompt vomiting and full recovery. In one worldwide review of cases over a ten-year period, there were thirty-eight episodes identified and sixteen deaths.[137]

In contrast, there were 205 deaths reported from paracetamol poisoning in Australia alone over a ten-year period from 2007-2017.[138]

There is almost no risk of harm from nicotine when vaping. Like smokers, vapers regulate their nicotine intake to maintain a comfortable nicotine level in the body. Exceeding the usual level rapidly produces nausea and a prompt reduction in use.

Nicotine liquid can be absorbed through the skin, but absorption is slow. Accidental spills over small areas of the fingers or hands in adults are highly unlikely to be a serious health concern and reported cases of harm are extremely rare.[139] Nevertheless, it is sensible to use gloves when handling highly concentrated nicotine liquid (100mg/mL), to clean up spills promptly and to wash your hands after handling nicotine.

What about fires and explosions?

Lithium-ion batteries in vaporisers can malfunction resulting in burns and traumatic injuries.[140] Malfunctions of this type do not occur in the popular beginner models (i.e. pod devices and pen-style models) because the battery is sealed inside the casing. Most problems occur with loose, replaceable batteries and unregulated 'mechanical mods' which have been used incorrectly.

Lithium-ion battery malfunctions also occur in other electrical devices such as mobile phones and laptops.[141]

There have been reports of vaping products causing fires. However, many more fires are caused by cigarettes. Most incidents could be prevented by user education. See Part 2 for more about vaping safely.

Peter

Peter first consulted me in 2015 when he was forty-one years old. He started smoking at fifteen years of age and had smoked forty to fifty cigarettes a day for twenty-five years.

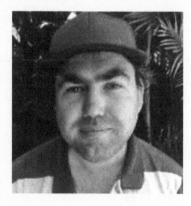

Peter was on the Disability Support Pension then due to mental health problems. Out of his $400 weekly pension, he was spending $280 per week on cigarettes and $115 on rent and had a huge credit card bill.

At our first meeting he told me, 'Smokes have been my best friend since I was a kid. I always turn to them when times are bad.' He tried to stop smoking many times with patches and lozenges, but always relapsed when under stress. Last time he gained five to ten kilograms.

I prescribed high-dose nicotine replacement. At one stage he was on two full strength nicotine patches and twenty 4mg lozenges per day. He got a rash from the patch but still smoked. Adding a cigalike (see page 94) helped a little, but he didn't have enough 'throat hit' and he still couldn't quit completely.

In July 2016 Peter started using a stronger vaping device, a vape pen with 18mg/mL nicotine e-liquid and quit smoking immediately. He said at the time, 'It's more satisfying than a cigarette.'

He had one brief lapse when his e-liquid supply was delayed but has otherwise not smoked for five years.

Since quitting smoking, Peter has saved many thousands of dollars, paid off his credit card bill and has more money to spend on food and taxis. He has not gained any weight since quitting and weighs two kilograms less than when I first met him. He is breathing better, has more energy and is coping better with stress. His sleep apnoea has also improved, and he is sleeping better.

Peter said to me 'I never thought I'd be able to quit. It's the best thing I've ever done. I prefer the e-cigarette to smoking. The e-cigarette helps me manage the bad days.'

He stopped using nicotine in mid-2019 and quit vaping altogether a few months later.

5

IS VAPING AN EFFECTIVE QUITTING AID?

Take-home messages

- Vaping is an evidence-based quitting aid
- It is more effective than nicotine replacement therapy in helping smokers quit
- Smoking rates are falling much faster in countries where vaping is readily accessible
- There are currently 68 million vapers world-wide

Vaping is not a 'silver bullet', but there is growing evidence that it helps many smokers to quit. Vaping with nicotine is more effective than using nicotine replacement therapy (nicotine patch, gum, lozenge, spray or inhalator).

In its 2021 report, the UK College of Physicians concluded, 'E-cigarettes are an effective treatment for tobacco dependency and their use should be included and encouraged in all treatment pathways.'[142]

The evidence for vaping comes from several different types of scientific studies including

- Randomised controlled trials

- Observational studies
- Population studies
- Trends in national smoking rates in countries where vaping nicotine is legal and accessible

Each type of evidence has its strengths and weaknesses. Combining results from different types of research (known as 'triangulation') provides a more accurate picture than relying on just one type of evidence.[143] Triangulation increases the confidence that vaping is an effective quitting aid.

Randomised controlled trials

'Randomised controlled trials' (RCTs) are the best way to test whether a medicine or treatment works. In these studies, half of the subjects are randomly allocated to use a nicotine vaping device and the other half use a different method of quitting in a controlled research setting. Any difference in the quit rates between the groups at the end of the study (usually at least six months after starting) reflects the difference in the effectiveness of the treatments. The RCTs so far suggest that vaping nicotine is 50-100% more effective than nicotine replacement therapy. Further trials are needed to strengthen the confidence in these findings.

Randomised controlled trials

Large studies

A study of 886 English smokers compared vaping with nicotine replacement therapy (NRT).[108] Half the subjects were given a vaping device with nicotine e-liquid and the other half used nicotine patches, gum or a combination of NRT products. After twelve months, twice as many smokers in the vaping group had quit smoking compared to the nicotine replacement group.

Another study of 1,800 New Zealand smokers found that adding vaping nicotine to a nicotine patch tripled the success rate after six months compared to using the patch alone.[144]

Pooled analyses

A Cochrane review is a high-quality, independent analysis which combines the best quality research studies of a particular treatment to assess whether it works. The most recent Cochrane review of four studies (September 2021) concluded that vaping with nicotine liquid was 53% more effective than nicotine replacement in helping smokers quit.[145] This means that out of 100 smokers, 6 will quit with NRT and 9 will quit with vaping nicotine.

Two other recent analyses concluded that vaping was 69% more effective than NRT[146, 147] and a third review of seven studies by Australian academics determined that it was 49% more effective.[148]

Two other analyses of RCTs concluded that vaping is no more effective than NRT.[149, 150] However, both contained a study of vaping which did not use nicotine and should not have been included.[151]

A further analysis of nine RCTs which also included this flawed study found that smokers using vaping products were still 55% more likely to quit than those using conventional therapies.[152]

Older studies used early vaping products and were less convincing because they had unreliable batteries and delivered low nicotine levels. However, vape technology has improved considerably over the last decade. Studies with modern vaping products show they are more effective for quitting than earlier models.[153, 154]

Comparison to stop-smoking medicines

The evidence so far suggests that vaping nicotine is the single most effective quitting aid, more successful than all other smoking medications, including varenicline and bupropion.

Although no trials have directly tested vaping against these medicines, their effectiveness can be compared by analysing all the randomised controlled trials available using a special technique called a 'network meta-analysis'.

A network meta-analysis of 171 RCTs was recently carried out by the prestigious UK National Institute for Health Research, funded by the UK Department of Health and Social Care.[419] It found that vaping nicotine produced the best quit rates.

The order of effectiveness for the treatments was

1. Vaping nicotine (most effective)
2. Varenicline (Champix/Chantix)
3. Nicotine replacement therapy (patches, gum, lozenges etc)
4. Bupropion (Zyban/Wellbutrin) (least effective)

Further trials directly comparing vaping with the other medications are needed to confirm this finding.

Other evidence

RCTs are performed in a controlled research environment and only tell part of the story.[155] We also need to know whether vaping works in the real world, where its uptake and use is influenced by the appeal of the product to the smoker, price, community attitudes and public messaging.

Community studies also pick up 'accidental quitters', smokers who tried vaping without intending to quit and stopped smoking as a result, like Joe Hildebrand and Senator Hollie Hughes (see pages 8, 22). [156, 157] Accidental quitting does not occur with other methods such as NRT. Furthermore, some smokers in the community go through a long transition from smoking to vaping after trying different devices, flavours and vaping techniques. These quitters are not included as successes in clinical trials, as the follow up is often too short.

Observational studies

Real world (observational) studies also indicate that vaping is an effective quitting aid.

These studies follow smokers who try vaping and compare them to other smokers who do not vape. Observational studies are prone to bias and can produce misleading results. However, two reviews of the better-quality observational studies found that vaping nicotine significantly increased the chances of quitting smoking.[158, 159]

Population studies

Research in large populations has demonstrated that smokers who vape have higher quit rates than smokers who don't vape.

Two large US studies found that smokers who used a vaping device were 70% more likely to quit than those who did not vape.[160, 161] A large study of smokers in the UK also demonstrated that smokers who vaped had significantly higher quit rates than non-vapers.[162] This study also estimated that over 50,000 additional smokers stopped smoking in the UK with a vaping product in 2017 who would otherwise have carried on smoking.

Daily vaping is even more effective. In studies in the US, vapers who used their device every day were three to eight times more likely to quit than smokers who did not vape.[153, 163]

Trends in national smoking rates

The decline in smoking rates has accelerated in countries where vaping nicotine is encouraged compared to countries where it is restricted.

For example, the adult smoking rate in England has fallen three times faster than in Australia since 2013 when vaping started becoming popular. Since 2013, 25% fewer people smoke in England compared to an 8% decline in Australia.[164] It is highly likely that vaping has been a major contributor to this rapid decline.[142]

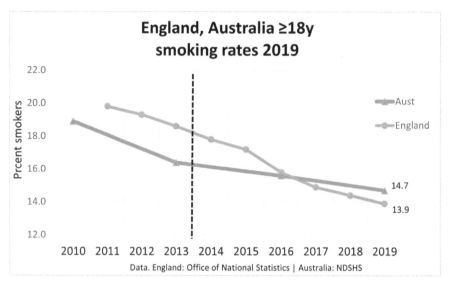

Decline in adult smoking in Australia and England since 2010

Restricting vaping increases smoking

Two studies in the US examined what happens when access to vaping is restricted. Both studies found that teen smoking increased significantly in states which banned the sales of vapes to young people compared to states without such bans.[165, 166] These studies suggest that vaping is a substitute for smoking. Simply, if more people vape, fewer will smoke.

National modelling studies

Modelling studies can be used to estimate the effect of vaping on national smoking rates by comparing the predicted decline in national smoking rates (without vaping) against the actual decline after vaping became available. Studies in England and the US both showed significant declines in smoking rates during the vaping era (2012-2018/19) compared to pre-vaping times.[167,168] The additional reduction in smoking rates attributed to vaping was 10% in the US and 20% in England. Reductions were greatest for the eighteen-to-thirty-five-year age groups who have most to gain from switching.

Testimonials

Further support comes from the many testimonials from former smokers who now vape and from those who no longer smoke or vape, including the cases in this book. You can read thousands more at www.righttovape. org. There are now an estimated 68 million people vaping globally.[29] While these testimonials and statistics are not scientific evidence, they should not be ignored.

Large population impact

The impact of a quitting aid at a population level depends on both its effectiveness and its reach (the number of people who use it). Vaping nicotine is an effective quitting method and is also the most popular quitting aid in Australia[5] and other western countries.[6-8] Vaping is an appealing option and smokers want to use it.

This combination gives vaping nicotine the potential to reduce smoking rates more than any other currently available option.

Easing restrictions on vaping in Australia would increase its uptake. One study estimated that making vaping as accessible in Australia as it is in the UK could save the lives of 645,000 current Australian smokers.[164]

Vaping may help prevent relapse to smoking

Every smoker knows that quitting is hard but staying quit is even harder. Half of all smokers who have quit for six months start smoking again and no treatments have been shown to prevent relapse.[169]

However, vaping may help to prevent relapse after quitting. According to the UK Royal College of Physicians,[142] 'A unique role of e-cigarettes in preventing relapse is emerging from UK qualitative research.' [10, 170]

Canadian guidelines also state 'Continued use of e-cigarettes may reduce risk of relapse to combustible tobacco.'[87]

This could be because vaping is a pleasurable substitute for smoking and helps the former smoker cope with urges to smoke. Most vapers say that they enjoy vaping more than smoking and find the smell and taste of smoking repugnant after vaping fruit and sweet flavours, reducing the risk of relapse.[10, 171]

Dianne

Dianne is a software developer and was a lifelong smoker who thought she would never be able to quit. She finally quit with vaping eight years ago at the age of sixty-three.

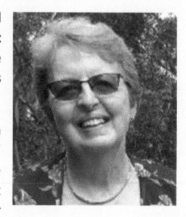

Dianne started smoking secretly when she was thirteen in the 'chook shed' at home and was soon hooked. She smoked heavily every day of her adult life, even unable to stop during her two pregnancies.

Dianne tried 'cold turkey', nicotine gum and patches with no success.

'I could never imagine a time when I would actually stop. I enjoyed it too much,' she told me. 'I was going to be a smoker when I died. I saw myself outside a hospital in the rain, wearing a hospital gown and dragging my drip with me, as I went for another desperate cigarette.'

In 2012, she developed a 'horrible, horrible hacking cough that went on and on and never went away.' At three p.m. on Friday 28 June 2013 she decided to give vaping a go.

'To my surprise, I quit instantly. I have never had a cigarette since that day and have never craved a cigarette.' That was almost eight years ago.

Dianne puts this success down to the fact that vaping mimics the hand-to-mouth action of smoking, but she was also very addicted to nicotine.

'My sense of smell returned within a couple of weeks. The cough disappeared after some months and has not come back. I don't smell and I feel a lot better.'

She started with a cigalike but quickly progressed to a vape pen with 18mg/mL nicotine. She now uses an advanced squonker device with 6mg/mL nicotine, mixing her own fruit/menthol flavoured juice.

'I still vape, but I am becoming less dependent on it. I can forget to take my vape with me when I go shopping and NOT drive back home to get it. I hope to eliminate nicotine completely over the next couple of years and hope to eventually stop vaping entirely.'

Dianne's advice to smokers is to 'seek out a helpful vape shop and give vaping a try. For me it was a lifesaver.'

PART 2

Start Vaping

So, you have decided to stop smoking and give vaping a try. Great! If you can't quit with conventional treatments, switching to vaping nicotine is the best thing you will ever do for your health.

This section provides practical information about vaping to help you in your discussions with your GP. Discuss with your GP whether vaping is appropriate for you and, if so, which device and e-liquid you should purchase. Nicotine vaping products can only be obtained with a prescription from your GP or another medical practitioner and it is illegal in Australia to vape nicotine without one.

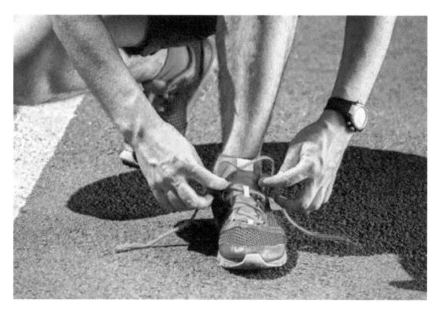

Let's get started!

6

DO YOUR HOMEWORK

Take-home messages

- Find out as much as you can about vaping before you jump in
- Vape shop staff provide expert advice on vaping, what to buy, instructions on correct use, safety issues and ongoing support
- Online forums, Facebook groups, educational websites and online reviewers provide valuable information
- Discuss vaping with your doctor

You can get a lot of useful information about vaping from vape shop staff, other vapers, online forums, Facebook groups and reddit.[171,172] There is also a wealth of other online information, including blogs and YouTube videos. Some simple advice at the start can point you in the right direction and prepares you for discussion with your GP and your first purchase.

Vape shops

Australian brick-and-mortar vape shops are modern-day quit clinics and are a valuable resource for both beginners and experienced vapers. Specialist vape shops are almost entirely owned and staffed by former smokers who now vape and genuinely want to help other smokers quit.

While the decision as to whether you should start vaping nicotine should be made in consultation with your doctor, vape shops can provide helpful information about the devices and e-liquids. They can show you how to operate the device, fill it correctly and use it safely. They provide support and advice over time and help with troubleshooting when problems arise.

Many vape shops provide a social and supportive environment for vapers with the opportunity to meet and speak with like-minded people.[173] Many vapers appreciate the sense of community and emotional support that vape shops offer.

Vape shop customers report high rates of successfully quitting smoking. In one study in Italy, 41% of first-time vape shop visitors were not smoking twelve months later.[174] Smokers who purchase vaporisers from vape shops are more successful in quitting smoking than those who purchase them online or at other retail outlets.[174,175]

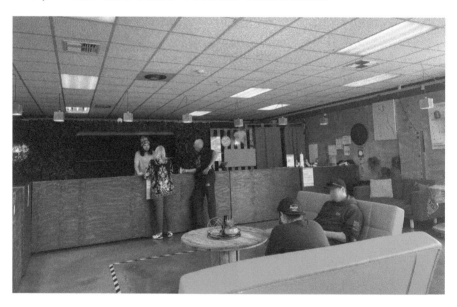

A vape shop in Adelaide

Online resources

A wide range of resources is available online to help new vapers. A full list is available in the Appendix. They include

Online forums	Forums are friendly support and discussion groups where new vapers can ask questions and share information e.g., Vaping in Australia, https://vapinginaustralia.com/
Facebook groups	A range of Australian Facebook groups are available to support new vapers. Some specialise in specific interests such as DIY juice mixing or pod devices and there is a group for women e.g., Vape Fam Australia, https://www.facebook.com/groups/2970172996629644
ATHRA	Australian Tobacco Harm Reduction Association (ATHRA) is an independent Australian health promotion charity providing extensive evidence-based information on vaping www.athra.org.au
Government websites	New Zealand and UK government websites are reliable and authoritative New Zealand, https://vapingfacts.health.nz/ UK, https://www.nhs.uk/smokefree
Websites	Several excellent commercial websites provide blogs, reviews and advice for beginners e.g., Vaping360, https://vaping360.com/
Reviewers	Vaping experts produce regular YouTube videos about vaping news, reviews and advocacy e.g., Legion Vapes (Steve), https://www.youtube.com/legionvapes

Health professionals

Speak to your GP about your smoking and whether vaping is appropriate for you. Some GPs can give good advice on vaping. They can also provide additional counselling and support which can improve success rates.

However, other GPs are uncertain about vaping. Australian health and medical organisations have taken an overly cautious view of vaping and this has created doubt for health professionals about its safety and effectiveness. Research shows that GPs rarely raise the subject of vaping on their own and recommend it even less often.[176, 177]

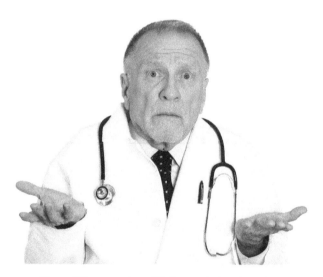

Many GPs are not well informed about vaping

Health professionals knowledge of vaping is 'largely derived from media, advertising, internet, newspaper articles and patient experience,' not from medical journals or professional sources, according to an Australian study.[177] However, some training in vaping is now beginning to be made available.

If you have successfully stopped smoking by switching to vaping, be sure to tell your doctor about it. The more they hear this, the better informed they will be.

The media

The mainstream media is not generally a reliable source of information on vaping and has contributed to the widespread misperceptions. An analysis of media reports of vaping found that it was unbalanced, focusing more on the risks of vaping and far less on the substantial health benefits.[31] Media reports favour negative and alarmist stories, often exaggerate risks and sometimes misrepresent scientific evidence. It is no wonder that the public is highly misinformed about vaping.

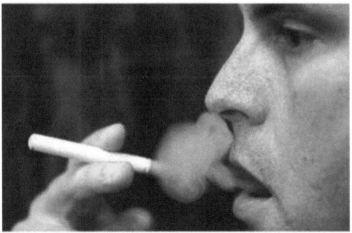

Media reports are often alarmist and exaggerate risks

Evidence of harm from vaping, including 'junk science' is reported enthusiastically. However scientific corrections of flawed reports get very little attention. Cancer Research UK responded after some disturbing and inaccurate media stories, explaining that 'headlines saying vaping might cause cancer are wildly misleading'[178] and published '6 tips to spot cancer fake news'.[179]

The role of the media is discussed further in Part 3.

Steve

Steve is a fifty-three-year-old former smoker from Lismore, NSW. Switching to vaping was a life-changing experience for him. He now runs a YouTube channel 'devoted to vaping and knowledge.'

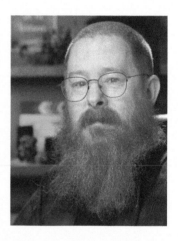

Steve smoked a full pack a day for three decades. 'I never wanted to quit smoking. I enjoyed it too much. Smoking was my best friend. No matter how bad things were, I could always have a smoke. Lose a job? Have a smoke to commiserate. Have a great day at work? Have a smoke to celebrate. In fact, the first thing I did when I heard that my mother had died of lung cancer was go sit in the backyard and smoke.'

However, Steve realised that this 'friend' was toxic and tried to quit repeatedly. 'Patches, lozenges, gums and self-help books. I tried them all and subconsciously sabotaged every effort. Even when I started to feel the early signs of emphysema ... wheezing, whistling, bubbling chest ... even then I resigned myself to an early death, clutching a pack of ciggies.'

Then one day he stumbled across vaping and started with a little sub-ohm device and some vanilla e-liquid. 'I instantly recognised that this could work if I let it. It promised to replace all the things

I loved about smoking while taking away or reducing all the things that were a problem.'

'I've been vaping for five years now and haven't had a cigarette since I started. In fact, I haven't even felt tempted. I enjoy the range of flavours and different styles of devices. Those early signs of emphysema went away, my breathing is now free and clear. No more whistling when I lay down.'

'I thought I would never be able to quit. My life was so profoundly changed by this that I dedicated myself to education and advocacy.'

Steve runs a highly informative and entertaining YouTube channel at https://www.youtube.com/legionvapes. Please check it out.

7

COILS, BATTERIES, CHIPSETS AND VAPING STYLES

Take-home messages

- Every vape has a metal heating coil to vaporise the e-liquid
- The 'electrical resistance' of the coil determines the performance of the device and cloud production
- Coils need replacement every one to four weeks except in cigalikes, disposables and some pod devices
- Built-in lithium-ion batteries are safer and easier to use than removable batteries
- The chipset in every 'regulated' vape device ensures safe operation and regulates the vaping process
- Most beginners start with a 'mouth-to-lung' device

When you start vaping, there is a whole new language to learn. There is a glossary of vaping terms in the Appendix to help make sense of it all. It is also helpful to know more about some of the key components of vaporisers before you go to the vape shop.

Coils, wicks and atomisers

The 'coil' is the metal heating element at the heart of each vaping device. When you breathe in or press the fire button, electricity from the battery flows through the coil, which in turn heats and vaporises the e-liquid.

The coil is located in the pod or tank of e-liquid. It is surrounded by a wick made of soft, absorbent material, usually cotton. The cotton wick draws e-liquid onto the coil. The coil and wick are usually inside a metal casing with holes to allow liquid inside. The whole unit is known as an 'atomiser'. However, in practice, the term coil and atomiser are used interchangeably.

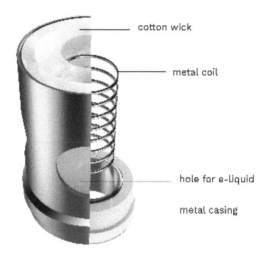

cotton wick

metal coil

hole for e-liquid

metal casing

Anatomy of an atomiser

There are two popular types of coils. The standard one is a single thread of metal wire coiled into a spiral shape. A more recent variation is the mesh coil, essentially a strip of metal with holes punched in it. Mesh coils have a larger surface area and heat more quickly. They produce a more intense flavour and larger clouds of vapour. They also last longer between coil changes.

Coils are usually made from 'nichrome' (chromium and nickel) or 'kanthal' (iron, chromium and aluminium) but also from nickel, titanium and stainless steel.

Coil resistance

The electrical resistance of a coil indicates how much it 'resists' the electrical current flowing through it. More current flows through low resistance coils. Resistance is measured in ohms (Ω) and most coils are between 0.05-3.5 Ω.

- Higher resistance coils (typically >1 Ω) are used for 'mouth-to-lung' vaping (see page 77). They use less power and produce smaller and cooler clouds.
- Low resistance coils (typically <1 Ω) use more power and are used for direct-to-lung vaping, generating larger, warmer clouds. This is also known as 'sub-ohming' as the coil resistance is sub (under) 1 Ω.

Some devices come with both low and high resistance coils so you can select how you want to vape.

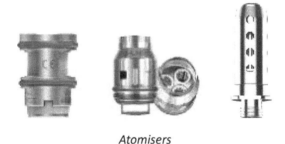

Atomisers

When to change a coil

Coils burn out over time and need to be replaced at regular intervals. This is typically every one to four weeks, depending on how heavily you vape, the power you use and the type of coil. Sweet flavours also reduce coil life.

You do not need to change coils in pre-filled pod vapes or disposables. The pod or disposable are discarded after a single use.

Signs that you may need a new coil are a change or reduction in flavour, reduced vapour production or a burnt taste. Burnt coils can also cause your tank to leak.

It is especially important to avoid vaping on an empty tank. The hot coil will burn the cotton wick and overheat any remaining e-liquid, delivering a cocktail of horrible tasting toxic chemicals known as a 'dry hit'.

If your device uses replaceable coils, it is important to always have spare coils handy, along with some spare juice.

How to change a coil

To change the coil in most models, you need to take the device apart and drain the liquid. Check your user manual or speak to the vape shop staff if you need help. Here are some general guidelines:

- Unscrew and remove the tank from the battery compartment while holding it upside down
- Pull out the old coil from the base of the tank
- Empty the tank (most models)
- Prime your new coil by adding one or two drops of e-liquid onto the cotton wick through each hole. Most coils have several holes on the outside. This allows you to start vaping faster, within a few minutes
- Twist the new coil into place
- Screw the tank back onto the battery
- Refill the tank with e-liquid
- Wait five minutes after filling the tank for the wick to saturate before you start vaping

Some newer pod models allow you to simply pull the old coil out from the base of the pod and replace it with a new one, without having to empty the tank.

Some vaping enthusiasts 'build' (make) their own coils and wicks to save money and for better performance.

Batteries

Almost all vaporisers are powered by one or more lithium-ion batteries. The battery supplies electricity to heat the coil to convert the e-liquid into an aerosol. Lithium-ion batteries are also used in many other consumer goods, such as mobile phones, laptop computers and even electronic cars.

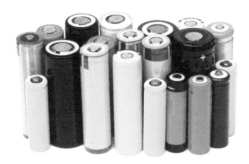

Different types of lithium-ion batteries

The capacity of the battery is measured in mAh (milliamp hours) and indicates how long it can last on a single charge. Batteries range from 200-300 mAh in cigalikes to 3500 mAh or more in larger devices.

A number of different lithium-ion batteries are used for vaping. Model 18650 is the most popular and has a long history of safe and reliable use. The number tells you it is 18mm high and 65mm long. A single 18650 can deliver up to 3500 mAh and has a lifespan of about 300-500 charging cycles.

Models 21700, 20700 and 26650 are larger and more powerful. They last longer between charges but are slower to charge. Always use the battery that is recommended for your device.

Built-in or removable batteries?

The batteries of most starter models such as pod devices, vape pens and disposables, are sealed inside the casing and are not removable. Models with built-in batteries are safer and simpler to use and are better for beginners.

More advanced devices use removable batteries which can be taken out and charged in an external battery charger. The advantage of removable batteries is that you can take a spare battery with you in case you run out of power. Also, batteries have a limited life. If the battery dies, you can just replace the battery and not the whole device.

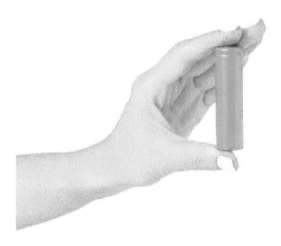

Model 18650 battery

Batteries differ in quality. If you are using removable batteries, it is important to buy good quality brand-name batteries from a vape shop and to be sure it is suitable for your device. Not all lithium-ion batteries are rated for high current applications like vaping and are at-risk of over-heating or even catching fire.

You can also find out more from Mooch, the vaping community's expert on batteries and electronics, here: www.facebook.com/batterymooch.

Chipsets

A chipset (an integrated circuit) is the 'brains' of every 'regulated' vaping product and is responsible for the safe operation of the device.

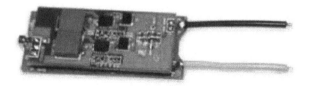

A chipset for a vaporiser

The chipset helps to maintain electrical safety and protects the device from overheating. It cuts out the power if there is a malfunction or if the fire button is pressed for too long. It can also prevent overcharging of batteries.

More advanced devices such as box mods and pod mods have sophisticated chipsets which allow you to control and adjust the power (wattage) or temperature of your device. They ensure the right amount of power is delivered to the coil to maintain an even performance.

The chipset in advanced devices also monitors settings such as power, voltage, coil resistance, coil temperature, battery charge remaining and the number of puffs, and displays them on an LED screen.

However, chipsets are not infallible and other safety guidelines should always be followed.

Vaping styles

The great majority of vapers start with mouth-to-lung vaping, but what on earth does this mean?

Mouth-to-lung (MTL) is the familiar two-stage inhalation style that most smokers use. You first draw the smoke into your mouth and then inhale into the lungs as a second step. When you start vaping it is best to begin with the same technique as smoking to make the transition to vaping easier.

Mouth-to-lung devices have a tighter draw like a cigarette and produce smaller, more discreet clouds of vapour. All the devices described in this book are suitable for mouth-to-lung vaping, including the advanced ones.

Direct-to-lung (DTL) is a different way of breathing in, preferred by some vapers and used by waterpipe smokers. Direct-to-lung vaping (or 'sub-ohming') means taking a deep breath directly into the lungs in one movement, like inhaling before diving into water. The clouds produced are much bigger and warmer and the flavour is stronger. DTL vaping has a greater health risk because it generates larger clouds at high temperatures with more toxic chemicals.[180]

Discuss DTL vaping with the vape shop staff if mouth-to-lung vaping does not suit you.

This table outlines the differences between the two vaping styles:

	Mouth-to-lung	Direct-to-lung
Similarity to smoking	Same technique as smoking	Different to smoking
Draw	Tighter, like a cigarette	Looser and airier
Coil used	High resistance, generally >1 Ω	Low resistance, generally <1 Ω
Power (wattage)	Low power devices	Higher power devices
Clouds	Small, cooler, less flavour	Large, warmer, fuller flavour
Nicotine concentration	Higher	Lower, typically 3-6mg/mL
Liquid volume used	Smaller volumes	Larger volumes
PG:VG	Higher PG e-liquids	Higher VG e-liquids
Suitable devices	Disposables, cigalikes, pod vapes, some box mods and most vape pens	Some vape pens, most box mods and pod mods Many modern tanks are optimised for DTL vaping

Fiona Patten MP

Fiona is a Member of the Victorian Legislative Council and the founder and leader of the Reason Party. She is also a vaper.

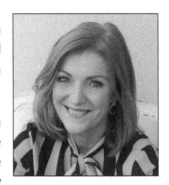

'I smoked when it was cool and Virginia Slims were the cigarette of choice in the Kensington Junior High girls' toilet. The tagline was 'you've come a long way baby', and well, yes, I have, because after smoking on and off for thirty years I no longer do.

I vape and that might make me a criminal in the federal Health Minister's eyes, but I am a healthier and happier one. I can now smell so much more but I no longer stink. My taste buds are re-emerging, and I no longer taste like the proverbial ashtray.

Like most of us I tried to give up the durries numerous times. I went 'cold turkey', I tried gum, I even tried the tampon shaped nicotine inhaler, but it was when someone introduced me to a vaporiser that I was able to give up permanently.

There are still times when I feel like smoking. It is generally when I am around smoking friends and wine is flowing. I think to myself, I could just have one … but I have lost count of the number of times that I have thought that and found myself a week later buying another pack. Now I pick up my vape and the moment passes. I use a small pre-filled 5% nicotine salt pod vape which does the trick for me.

I am still consuming nicotine but my desire for it is diminishing, and I suspect that there will be a time soon when I won't always have a vape in my handbag.

As someone who has been passionate about harm minimisation, I join the experts in attesting that vaping is not harmless, but it is a hell of a lot less harmful than smoking.

Now if we can just get the state and federal Health Ministers to listen to the experts I can cease being seen as a criminal for taking steps to look after my health.'

Fiona gave the keynote address on vaping at the Global Forum for Nicotine in 2021.

www.fionapatten.com.au

8

STARTER VAPE KITS

Take-home messages

- There is a wide range of devices from simple disposables to complex and powerful 'box mods'
- Selection is based on similarity to a cigarette, ease of use, nicotine delivery, device size, battery life and budget
- The most popular starter models are pod vapes (pre-filled and re-fillable) which are compact, easy-to-use and have good nicotine delivery
- Disposables, vape pens and cigalikes ('cigarette-like') are also suitable starter models
- Don't give up. You may need to try different products until you find the one that works best for you

There is a staggering range of vaporisers available so choosing your first vape can feel overwhelming! However, the wide choice means there is a device that is likely to suit your needs.

This chapter discusses starter devices which are recommended for beginners. All these devices will help to ease your transition from smoking to vaping with a minimum of fuss.

Don't be intimidated by the technology and scary terms like temperature control, mechanical mods and rebuildable dripping atomisers. There are many very easy-to-use and effective devices which do not require any technical knowledge.

If you like technology and want a more complex model, you may prefer to start with a more advanced device. These are discussed in Chapter 9.

No vaping devices have been approved by Australia's medicines regulator, the Therapeutic Goods Administration.

All vaporisers consist of two basic components which are joined together: a tank or pod which holds the coil and e-liquid, and a battery compartment.

Components	Cigalike	Pod vape	Vape pen	Box mod
Tank or pod • E-liquid • Coil • Mouthpiece • Variable airflow control				
Battery compartment • Rechargeable battery • Fire/power button • Chipset • Flow sensor • Digital screen • Control buttons • Some cigalikes have an LED light at the tip				

All vaping devices consist of two parts: a tank or pod and a battery compartment

It is not uncommon at the start of your vaping journey to try different products until you find the one that works best for you. Don't give up if your first choice is not quite right.

The following table shows the different types of vaping products that are currently available. Different vendors sell different models, so you may need to shop around if you are looking for a particular device.

Pod vapes

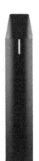

Prefilled pod vapes

- Most popular beginner model
- Very simple to use
- Good nicotine replacement
- Insert prefilled pod and discard pod when empty
- No filling, buttons, coil replacement or maintenance
- Rechargeable battery

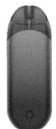

Refillable pod vapes

- Refill pod as needed
- Pod replaced when coil burns out
- Easy to use
- No coil replacement in most
- No settings to adjust
- Rechargeable battery

Other starter vapes

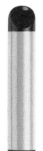

Disposables

- Very easy to use
- No filling, buttons, coil replacement or maintenance
- Good nicotine replacement (nicotine salt)

Cigalikes

- Looks and feels like a cigarette
- Very easy to use
- Replaceable cartomisers
- No filling, buttons, coil replacement or maintenance
- Modest nicotine replacement (freebase nicotine)
- Rechargeable battery

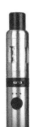

Vape pens

- Larger, pen shaped
- More complex to use
- Refillable tank
- Coil changes needed
- Rechargeable battery

Advanced models

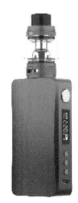

Box mods

- Larger and more complex
- Many features
- Highly customisable
- Refillable tank
- Coil changes needed
- Display screen
- Larger battery, more power and larger clouds
- Rechargeable battery

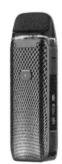

Pod mods

- Detachable, easy-to-fill pod
- Bigger battery, more power and longer lasting than pod vapes
- Customisable features
- Display screen
- Coil changes needed, but simplified
- Rechargeable battery

Range of vaping devices for beginners

The vaping product you choose depends on your personal preferences. Some of the issues to consider in selecting a device are listed in the following box. Don't be afraid to experiment until you find one you like.

Checklist for choosing a vaporiser

- What is your smoking style, mouth-to-lung or direct-to-lung?
- Do you want a device that looks and feels like a cigarette?
- Do you want a very easy-to-use device?
- Are you willing to replace coils and refill a tank?
- Do you want to make small or large clouds?
- Does size matter?
- Do you need a device that delivers high levels of nicotine?
- Do you want a built-in or removable battery?
- Do you need a long-lasting battery to get you through the whole day?
- What is your budget?

Pod vapes

Pod vapes are the most popular category for new vapers. All models consist of a detachable pod containing e-liquid and a rechargeable battery. There are two types of pod vapes: those with disposable pre-filled pods and others which use re-fillable pods.

1 Pre-filled pod vapes

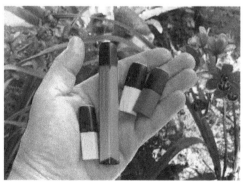

Pre-filled pod vape with replacement pods

Pre-filled pod vapes consist of a rechargeable battery and a sealed, disposable pod and are ideal for smokers making the switch to vaping. They are very easy to use and mimic the experience of smoking. Simply 'plug and play'.

Each pod contains a coil and is pre-filled with ready-to-use nicotine e-liquid. When the pod is empty, it is discarded and replaced with a new one. There is no need to refill the device with e-liquid or change the coil and there are no buttons or settings to adjust.

Importantly, pre-filled pod vapes provide a similar nicotine hit to a cigarette. They use nicotine salt in concentrations of 20-60mg/mL in a range of flavours. A pod of 50mg/mL nicotine salt contains about the same amount of nicotine as a pack of 20 cigarettes but this varies between brands.[181]

Each pod typically contains 1-2mL of e-liquid and delivers 200-300 puffs, equivalent to about one to one-and-a-half packets of cigarettes. The battery is generally 350-400 mAh capacity.

Research on nicotine salt pod devices show they have high success rates as a quitting aid. This is probably due to their ability to deliver nicotine like traditional cigarettes and to closely mimic smoking behaviour.[182]

Pods which are pre-filled with nicotine can be imported from overseas or purchased from participating Australian pharmacies with a prescription.

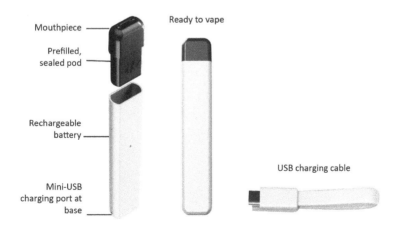

Mouthpiece

Prefilled, sealed pod

Rechargeable battery

Mini-USB charging port at base

Ready to vape

USB charging cable

Parts of a pre-filled pod device

Average cost

- Device and charging cable $30-40
- Pre-filled pods $7-10 each

Pros	Cons
Similar look and feel of a cigarette	Pods are relatively expensive
Very easy to use and maintain	Shorter battery life
No refilling or coil replacement	Limited range of flavours
Good nicotine delivery and 'throat hit'	Environmental impact from disposable pods
Compact and portable	
Discreet, small vapour clouds	
Safer for homes with small children	

2 Re-fillable pod vapes

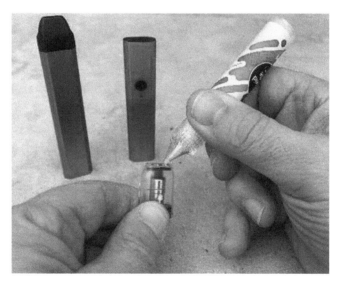

Refilling a pod

Re-fillable pod vapes have a reusable pod which you refill from a bottle of e-liquid. Each pod is re-used several times and replaced when the internal coil burns out, typically after 1-2 weeks.

Some models have replaceable coils, so you can keep using the pod and replace the coil when needed. Coils are easily replaced by slipping them out from the base of the pod, a much simpler process than replacing the coil in the 'tank' in more sophisticated devices.

Pods are generally filled via a small filling port on the outside of the pod.

Re-fillable pod models are larger than pre-filled pod devices with a larger rechargeable battery (650-1500 mAh) which lasts longer between charges. They are also cheaper to use as you can buy bottles of e-liquid rather than more costly individual pods.

Some models have a fire button which you press when inhaling while others are breath-activated (they turn on when you inhale). Re-fillable pod models typically put out 15-18W of power and have tanks from 2-3.5mL

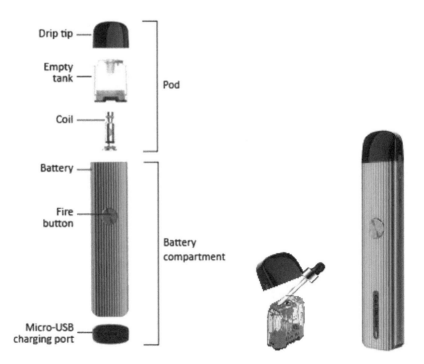

A re-fillable pod vape with a replaceable coil

Refillable pod vapes come in a wide range of shapes and sizes. Some are small and compact. Others are considerably larger.

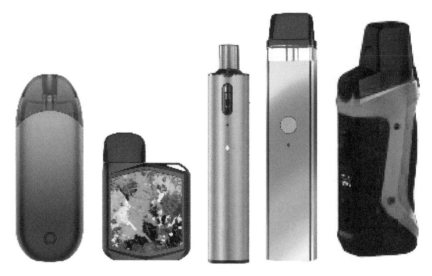

There is a wide variety of re-fillable pod devices

Average cost

- Re-fillable pod device and charging cable $30-60
- Premixed nicotine salt e-liquid, 30ml: $30-35
- Empty replacement pods: $5-7

Pros	Cons
Easy to use	Need to refill
Inexpensive to buy and cheap to use	Some models use replacement coils which are easy to install
Good nicotine delivery (nicotine salt)	Not as safe for homes with small children (bottles of liquid nicotine required)
Most are compact and portable	

Other starter vapes

1 Disposables

Disposables are ideal beginner devices for smokers who want to start with a simple, easy-to-use product with good nicotine delivery. Put the device in your mouth, puff it like a cigarette and throw it away (in the bin) when it stops working. There is no need to worry about pressing buttons, priming, charging or refilling.

Disposables are available in two concentrations of nicotine salt, 20-30mg/mL and 50-60mg/mL. The higher concentration delivers a strong nicotine hit and is a good replacement for the more nicotine-dependent smoker.

They come in a range of sizes. The larger models typically have a 6mL tank, a 1000mAh battery and deliver up to 1,500-2,000 puffs. Smaller models have 1.2mL tanks, 250mAh battery and deliver about 300 puffs.

Disposables are available in a range of flavours including tobacco flavour.

Disposables with nicotine can be imported from overseas or purchased from participating pharmacies with a prescription.

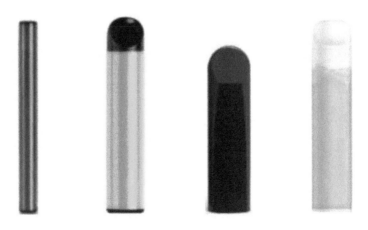

Disposable vapes

Average cost

- Large $25 each
- Small $10 each

Pros	Cons
Very simple and easy to use	More expensive
Good nicotine delivery	Greater environmental impact
Very compact and portable	Limited range of flavours
No maintenance. Discard after use	
Discreet, small vapour clouds	
Safer for homes with small children	

2 Vape pens

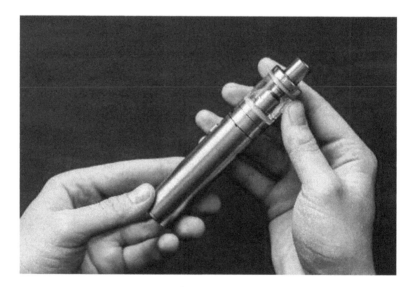

A vape pen

Vape pens are shaped like a pen or tube. They give good nicotine delivery but are more complex to use and maintain than pod vapes and disposables.

Vape pens have a 2-4 ml refillable tank which is topped up from a bottle of e-liquid, usually with freebase nicotine. (see page 117)

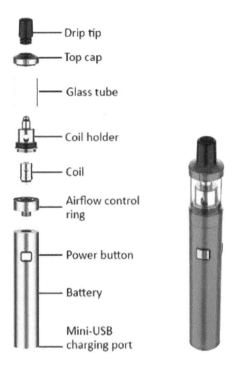

A vape pen - parts and complete device

The coil needs to be changed at regular intervals by taking the device apart and draining the e-liquid. Coil changing is a little fiddly and messy and may not appeal to some users.

The larger 1200-1500mAh battery lasts longer between charges than the battery in smaller models and makes larger clouds. Some vape pens have adjustable power and airflow settings as well.

Most vape pens are suited to mouth-to-lung vaping which is pre-ferred by most new vapers. Many models can also be used for direct-to-lung vaping by using a lower resistance coil and increasing the airflow.

Filling the tank

It is a good idea to refill your device when the liquid level in the tank gets down to a third or half. Vaping on an empty tank can lead to a burnt coil resulting in a foul tasting 'dry hit'.

The nicotine concentration used in vape pens is typically 3-24mg/mL freebase nicotine, although the higher levels can be harsh on the throat. Nicotine salt can be used instead for higher concentrations if preferred and is better tolerated.

Most vape pens are filled from the top, but some are filled from the bottom of the device. Check your manual to see what type you have and for filling instructions.

Top-fill tanks

Top-fill tanks are easier to fill as they do not have to be removed from the battery compartment. First, unscrew the top of the tank (or slide it to the side for some models). Slightly tilt your device at an angle and gently squeeze the e-liquid down the inside of the tank using a bottle with a dropper or fine tip. Avoid getting any e-liquid in the centre tube. Fill it up to the maximum fill line and avoid overfilling. Then screw or slide the top back on.

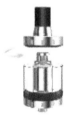 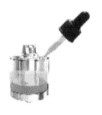 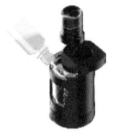

Removable mouthpiece: Unscrew the top of the tank, tilt and fill   *Sliding mouthpiece: Slide the top and fill*

Bottom-fill tanks

Unscrew the tank from the battery and remove the base of the tank to get access to the filing hole. Hold the tank at an angle and fill to the fill line. Make sure the e-juice does not enter the centre tube of the tank. Screw the base and reattach the tank to the battery unit. After refilling, wash any e-liquid from your hands.

Using a vape pen

Most vape pens are activated by pressing and holding the fire/power button as you inhale. Other models have no buttons and are breath-activated (simply breathe in). For models with adjustable power, you should start at a low power level (wattage) and gradually increase the power until you get the desired effect. Many models have airflow control so the draw can be tightened or loosened.

Changing the coil

The heating coil in a vape pen needs to be replaced at regular intervals, typically every one to four weeks. Ask the vape shop staff how to change the coil in your device and check your user manual.

Don't forget to always carry spare coils and e-liquid with you.

Average cost

- Vape pen: $35-60
- Replacement coils: $3-4 each
- Pre-mixed, flavoured, freebase nicotine e-liquid: 60ml $30-40 (lasts 12 days at 5ml per day)

Pros	Cons
Good nicotine delivery	More complex to maintain than closed systems: refilling and coil changes
Easy to use	Minimal customisation
Larger battery capacity	Not as safe for homes with small children
Very portable	
Inexpensive and cheap to use	
Larger vapour clouds	

3 Cigalikes

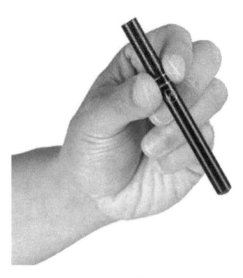

A cigalike

Cigalikes ('cigarette-like') look and feel like a traditional cigarette. They can be very effective for smokers who want to closely replicate the smoking ritual and sensations. They consist of

- A small, low-capacity, single-use battery, typically 170-300 mAh
- A cartomiser (a sealed reservoir of nicotine e-liquid with a heating coil)
- Some have a light at the tip which lights up when you inhale

Each cartomiser delivers a similar number of puffs to a packet or a pack and a half of cigarettes, typically 200-400 puffs depending on the brand. Most cigalikes use freebase nicotine in the 0-24mg/mL range and deliver only modest nicotine levels which may not be sufficiently strong for heavier smokers. They release relatively small, discreet clouds of vapour.

Some come with a portable charging case so you can recharge on the run. There is a range of flavours but the choice is limited by what the manufacturer provides.

Cigalikes are more expensive over the long-term due to the higher cost of purchasing the disposable cartomisers. Cigalike cartomisers with nicotine can be imported from overseas or purchased from participating Australian pharmacies with a prescription.

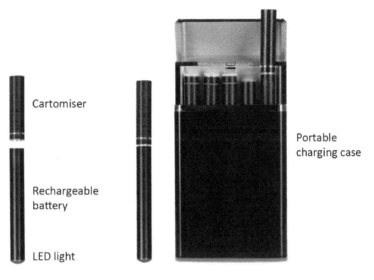

Cartomiser

Rechargeable battery

LED light

Portable charging case

Rechargeable cigalike with a portable charging case

Pros	Cons
Looks and feels like a traditional cigarette	Cartomisers are relatively expensive
Very easy to use and maintain	Modest nicotine delivery
No refilling or coil replacement	Limited range of flavours
Very compact and portable	Environmental impact from disposable cartomisers
Discreet, small vapour clouds	
Safer for homes with small children	

Rachael

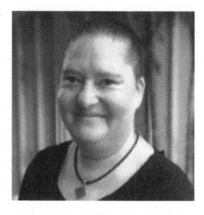

Rachael is a 39-year-old proudly Indigenous Wonnarua woman and is a former oncology (cancer) nurse from Newcastle who vapes.

Unfortunately, Rachael was forced to retire on the Disability Support Pension after a string of serious illnesses including rheumatoid arthritis, blood clots in the lung, endometriosis and depression. She lived alone and felt very isolated.

Rachael was smoking thirty to forty cigarettes a day for twenty years. She told me, 'As an oncology nurse I know how deadly smoking is and I didn't want to end up in the cancer ward as a patient. I'd tried practically everything to kick the habit over fifteen years.' Nicotine gum, lozenges, sprays, Champix, hypnosis, acupuncture … but nothing worked.

Two years ago, a family friend suggested vaping. She went to the local vape shop, bought her first pod and ordered some nicotine from overseas. 'Within days I was solely vaping, completely tobacco-free. I have been tobacco-free ever since, vaping custard, bakery and dessert flavours.'

'As someone with a background in health, I have read widely and thoroughly into vaping. I wouldn't vape if I wasn't personally satisfied with the risk I was taking.'

Rachael's health has improved dramatically over the last two years. 'I wake up in the morning able to breathe, and I'm not coughing up unbelievable amounts of junk. I'm less depressed, anxious, and suffer fewer panic attacks. I have more energy and stamina and my brain is working better. I find I can think more clearly.'

She has already saved thousands of dollars since quitting smoking. 'I struggled to manage financially on the pension. Now I can afford better food and can go out for a meal occasionally.'

Another benefit of vaping for Rachael was the support of the vaping community. 'I feel a sense of belonging, and have been accepted into a wonderful, supportive, amazing, helpful vaping family and community.'

Rachael has gradually reduced her nicotine intake and now is 'down to almost no nicotine.' She plans to quit vaping altogether in the future, and time will tell if she can.

9

ADVANCED MODELS

Take-home messages

- Some new vapers choose to start with a box mod or pod mod
- Box mods are larger and more complex and have a longer learning curve
- You can adjust the wattage, voltage and temperature and change parts of a box mod to customise your vaping experience
- Box mods have LED display screens, higher power output, high-capacity batteries and larger tanks
- The most suitable box mods for beginners are mouth-to-lung devices with a single built-in battery and moderate power
- Pod mods have the convenience of a removable pod but are less complex and powerful than box mods

It is generally best for beginners to become familiar with one of the starter models first as advanced models are more complex to operate. However, some new vapers do not find the starter models satisfying or prefer a device with more features.

The more advanced devices are called 'mods' because the settings and parts can be 'modified'. You can adjust the voltage, wattage and temperature to customise your vaping experience.

1 Box mods

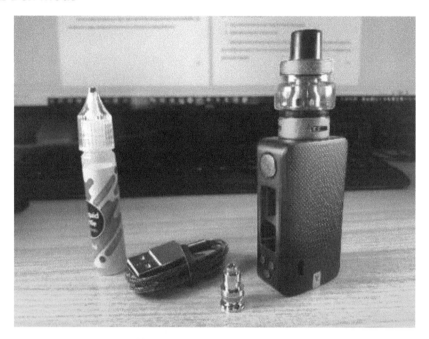

Box mod kit with spare coil and charging cable

The most popular mod devices are called 'box mods' and are box-like in shape. Box mods are more powerful than other devices and more complex to use. They have LED display screens, higher power output and high-capacity batteries. You can also change settings, tanks, batteries and other components.

Box mod vapes consist of two parts:

- A mod compartment which holds the battery and chipset
- A tank which holds the e-liquid and coil

Both parts can be purchased together as a 'kit' or individually. A kit is the best option for beginners as it is simple and ready to use. If you are buying the parts separately, make sure they are compatible and can be joined together.

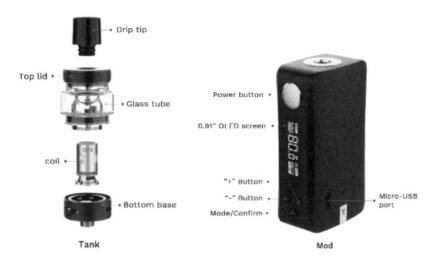

Parts of a box mod kit

Mods have refillable tanks and use replaceable coils which need changing. Most are designed for direct-to-lung sub-ohm vaping, producing bigger clouds and more intense sensations. However, some can also be used for mouth-to-lung vaping by using a higher resistance coil and reducing the airflow.

Box mods have larger batteries which deliver more power and last longer between charges. Some models have built-in batteries. Others use removable batteries which can be charged in an external battery charger. More powerful models have two to three or even four batteries.

The brain of a box mod is a sophisticated chipset which controls the operation of the device and regulates electrical safety.

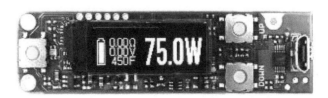

Printed circuit board with a chipset and display screen for a box mod

There are three main modes for controlling the performance of your mod:

- The most popular method is to vary the wattage. This involves setting the power in watts and adjusting it up or down until you achieve the desired effect. Higher power is used with low resistance coils to produce larger, warmer clouds with more flavour. The wattage can be adjusted by using the + and − control buttons or the touchscreen if there is one.

- Variable voltage is less popular and involves finding out the resistance of your coil and then setting an appropriate voltage to get the desired power output.

- Some box mods let you also set the temperature of the heating coil. Temperature control is a little more complicated and requires coils made of specific metals. It is much less popular than variable wattage.

Choosing a box mod

Suitable box mods for new vapers are models which can be used for mouth-to-lung vaping and have a single built-in battery. These devices have moderate (but sufficient) power up to 40W-80W.

Consider these issues when buying a box mod:

- Kits are a better choice for most beginners than buying a tank and box mod separately.

- Devices with built-in batteries are simpler and safer to use.

- The battery capacity for box mods typically varies from 1,000-3,000 mAh. Higher capacity batteries last longer between charges.

- Power up to a maximum output of 40-80W is more than adequate for most vapers, especially for mouth-to-lung use. Some direct-to-lung vapers may prefer a higher power level. Advanced models go up to 220W.

- Tanks vary from 2-8ml. The larger the tank, the less frequently it needs filling.

- How big is the display screen? Is it a touchscreen? Is it easy to read? Is the user interface easy to navigate?

- Size and bulk.

- Your budget.

Using a box mod

Using a box mod for the first time can be daunting. Check your manual for instructions and get advice from your local vape shop before starting. YouTube reviews of most models are available online and can be very helpful.

Here are some general guidelines to help get started:

Charge the battery	Fully charge the internal battery with the supplied cable. Removable batteries can be charged in the device or preferably removed and charged in an external battery charger.
Fill your device	Fill the tank with e-liquid. Check your manual for details.
	Most tanks are filled from the top. Take off the top of the tank (or slide it to the side for some models). Tilt the tank to one side and slowly squeeze the e-liquid down the side of the tank. Fill to the maximum fill line, avoiding getting any in the centre tube. Then screw the top back on. Allow at least five minutes for the wick to saturate before using a new coil.
	Bottom-fill tanks require a different filling technique.
	Top it up through the day when it gets to about one third full.

Turn it on

Most box mods are powered on by five clicks of the power button within two seconds or until the LED screen and indicator lights turn on.

You may also need to unlock the screen and buttons, usually by pressing two buttons simultaneously. Check the user manual for your device.

Adjust the settings

Most box mods allow you to vary the power (variable wattage) or temperature (temperature control). Settings can be changed using the control buttons or touchscreen. Some models have fixed settings and cannot be adjusted.

Access the menu, usually by pressing the power or mode button three times or via the touchscreen. Check your manual if this does not work.

Set the power in watts if using power control. The power setting depends on the coil being used. Check the manual or ask the vape shop staff what power you should start with for the coil you are using. Adjust your wattage and airflow until you get the vapour, flavour and throat hit you want. It is better to start low. Some devices will detect the coil resistance and set the wattage automatically.

If your device supports temperature control, you can set the coil temperature you want, usually between 200-250°C. Make sure you have the right coil type installed.

If your device has adjustable airflow, you can experiment to see if drawing in more or less air improves the experience.

Start vaping	Hold down the power button as you draw on the mouthpiece. Begin with a short puff and adjust your puffing until it feels right for you. Most devices cut off the power if you hold the button down too long to avoid burning the coil.
	If your device allows it, it is a good idea to lock your buttons and screen while vaping to avoid accidental changes. This is usually done by pressing two buttons simultaneously. Check the user manual for your device.
Turn it off	It is important to turn your device off after use to prevent accidental firing in your pocket or bag. Most box mods are powered off by five clicks on the power button in quick succession within two seconds.

Reading the display screen

Box mods have a sophisticated digital screen to display information such as:

- Power settings. The wattage is generally shown as a number followed by the letter 'W' for watts. Voltage is displayed with a number followed by 'V' for voltage. 'VW' indicates the device is in 'variable wattage' mode, and 'VV' indicates 'variable voltage' mode. Most vapers use variable wattage mode.

- The resistance of the coil indicated by the ohm symbol Ω, typically from 0.05 to 3.5 Ω.

- The battery charge remaining. The battery indicator is usually a battery symbol or a percentage.

- Temperature setting for devices with temperature control. TC indicates the device is in temperature control mode. The temperature is shown as a number followed by the letter 'C' for Celsius.

- A puff counter to measure the number of puffs you have taken and, in some models, the puff duration.

- Lock indicator.

- Error messages.

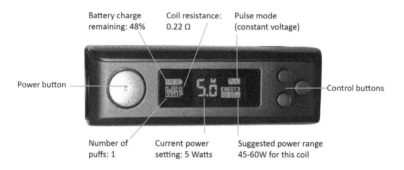

Simple non-touch screen with 3 control buttons

Coil replacement

The heating coil in a box mod needs to be replaced at regular intervals. Always make sure you have spare coils available.

Average cost

- Starter box mod kits with a single built-in battery and tank: $60-90 Larger devices with multiple external batteries and parts purchased separately are more costly

- Replacement coils: $3-6

Pros	Cons
Customisable settings and greater control over your vaping experience	Larger and bulkier
Longer battery life	More complex to use and maintain
Larger tanks for less frequent refilling	More expensive to purchase but cheaper to run

Good nicotine delivery and throat hit   Not as safe for homes with
small children

Larger clouds and more intense flavours

2 Pod mods

Pod mods are a popular half-way option between pod vapes and box
mods. They are hybrid devices which offer some of the convenience of
a pod vape and some of the more advanced features of a box mod in a
more compact size.

Pod mods consist of a mod (battery unit) with a detachable pod which
can be refilled a number of times and replaced when the coil burns out.
Many also use a replaceable coil, so the pod can be used for longer.

Compared to pod vapes, they have larger pods and batteries, greater
power, and can deliver more nicotine and larger clouds. Like box mods
they can be customised (e.g wattage and airflow) and have an LED screen
which displays the current settings.

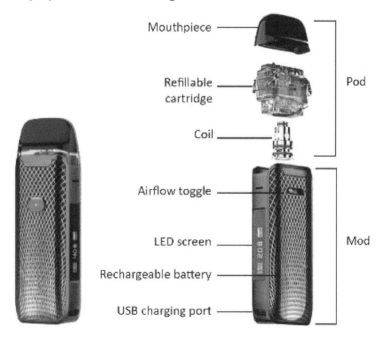

Mouthpiece

Refillable
cartridge   Pod

Coil

Airflow toggle

LED screen   Mod

Rechargeable battery

USB charging port

Parts of a pod mod

3 Unregulated mods

'Unregulated' mods are strictly for advanced users. These devices do not have a chipset and lack the standard safety features of regulated models and there is a higher risk of accidental injury. Users need to understand Ohm's law before using these devices.

- 'Mechanical mods' are used by some enthusiasts who want a powerful but simple device to produce large clouds. Pressing the power button connects the battery directly with the atomiser without electrical safety controls.
- 'Squonk mods' have a squeeze bottle of e-liquid in the battery compartment. The user squeezes e-liquid up into the atomiser to soak the wick before inhaling.

Which vaping device should you buy?

Buying a vaping device is a very personal decision. It depends on your own needs, budget and preferences for size and ease of use. Many people start with a simple pod vape or vape pen and some progress to a more advanced device over time. The table on the next page may help you decide.

Which vaping device is right for you?

	Cigalike	Disposable	Pre-filled Pod	Re-fillable pod	Vape pen	Pod mod	Box mod
Similarity to cigarette	Very similar	Very similar	Similar	Less similar	Quite different	Very different	Very different
Ease of use	Easy	Very easy	Easy	More complex	Complex	Very complex	Advanced users only
Size	Small	Small-medium	Small-medium	Small-medium	Medium	Medium	Large, bulky
E-liquid	Prefilled, replaceable cartridges	Prefilled disposable devices	Prefilled disposable pods	Pods refilled by the user	Refillable tank	Refillable pod	Refillable tank
Nicotine delivery	Mild	Moderate to high	Moderate to high	Moderate to high	Moderate to high	High	High
Modifiable	No	No	No	No	Partially	Moderately modifiable	Highly modifiable
Device cost	$	$	$$	$$$	$$$	$$$	$$$$
E-liquid cost	$$$	$$$	$$$	$	$	$	$

Hayley

Hayley is a 37-year-old stay-at-home mum from Perth with two 'very charismatic and energetic kids.' Her seven-year-old daughter has become a 'tiny advocate' for vaping.

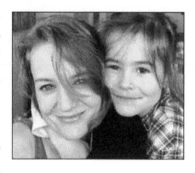

'In 2005, my boyfriend was in an accident in Thailand just weeks after the tsunami and sadly he died. At his funeral, a friend gave me a cigarette to settle me down. I smoked for the next thirteen years.

Over those years I tried Allen Carr books, hypnosis, Champix, patches and gums. None of these methods lasted more than a few weeks. I managed to abstain from cigarettes when I was pregnant with both of my children. But inevitably, stress and anxiety led to a relapse.

When my son was six months old, I knew I had to stop for good. I was living in the Netherlands where vaping is legal and encouraged, so my GP sent me to the local vape store in town. I started vaping and cigarettes were history. That was four years ago.

Since I switched to vaping, my asthma and migraines have greatly improved. I have what I call 'super-mum strength' to chase after my kids, carry my 17kg son around, lift furniture for restoration and am in general far more active than I was in my twenties. I owe it all to vaping and that GP who recommended it.

I started with a simple pen vape with strawberry flavour e-liquid and 18mg/mL nicotine. I then moved on to a box mod and quickly reduced my nicotine to 9mg/mL and now use a pod mod with 6mg/mL nicotine.

My seven-year-old daughter remembers when I smoked four years ago. She understands that I now vape instead of smoking and what's really great is that she is a tiny advocate for the cause. When we are out and she sees somebody smoking she will say "Mummy, you should tell that person about vaping. They will feel better just like you!"'

When Hayley's children are at school, she restores and refinishes furniture artistically. See her work at www.instagram. com/hayleys_suite_pieces

10

WHICH E-LIQUID?

Take-home messages

- All e-liquids are made from propylene glycol and/or vegetable glycerine. Nicotine and flavourings are optional.
- You may need nicotine if you are dependent on it from smoking or if you benefit from its positive effects such as improved concentration.
- You may not need nicotine if you are only smoking for the habit and the familiar ritual.
- Nicotine salt is smoother and quicker to act than freebase nicotine and can be used in higher doses.
- Nicotine salt is generally used in low-powered devices, such as small pod models and disposables.
- Start with a nicotine concentration based on your nicotine dependence and what device you are using.
- Most vapers start with tobacco flavour and switch to fruit, dessert, mint or other flavours later.
- Beginners usually purchase pre-mixed e-liquid with nicotine already added.
- Some experienced users add their own nicotine to flavoured e-liquid or mix their own e-liquids from scratch.

Having chosen your vaping device, your next task is to find the right e-liquid. E-liquid consists of four ingredients: nicotine (optional), flavourings (optional), propylene glycol (PG) and vegetable glycerine (VG).

Do you need nicotine? Should you get nicotine salt or freebase? What nicotine concentration do you need? What flavour should you start with? Premixed liquids or mix your own? Let's find out ...

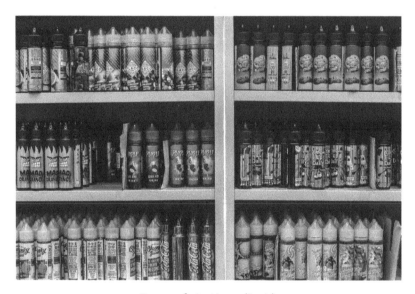

Range of nicotine e-liquids

Nicotine

Nicotine from vaping replaces the nicotine you crave from smoking. Nicotine also contributes to the familiar 'throat hit' (the sensation at the back of the throat when you inhale) which is part of the smoking experience.

Are you nicotine-dependent?

Most smokers have a physical dependence on nicotine. They suffer cravings for nicotine and feel irritable, anxious and have trouble sleeping without it.

Others hanker for nicotine because it improves their concentration, alertness, weight control, anxiety or mood. Nicotine also benefits some medical conditions such as schizophrenia, Parkinson's disease, ulcerative colitis and attention deficit hyperactivity disorder (ADHD).

However, not all vapers need nicotine. Some simply enjoy the ritual and sensations of smoking and vaping. Signs that the habit is important for you include:

- You enjoy the hand-to-mouth action and the sensations and tastes of smoking.

- You get strong urges to smoke at times of stress, with a drink, with friends, after dinner or from other smoking triggers.

- You enjoy a cigarette break as 'time out' or as a pause after a task.

- Smoking helps you socialise and connect with other people or when you are bored.

- You identify as a smoker. Smoking is part of who you are. You may feel smoking is a friend and helps you cope with life and difficult times.

If your smoking is mainly driven by habit, you may need less nicotine or possibly none at all. Simply replicating the smoking ritual by vaping at times when you would normally smoke may be the key for you.

You can calculate your nicotine dependence with two questions:

- How many cigarettes do you smoke daily? The more you smoke, the more heavily dependent you are likely to be on nicotine.

- How long after you wake up in the morning do you have your first cigarette? The nicotine level in your body drops dramatically overnight and you wake craving a cigarette. The earlier you have the first cigarette of the day after waking, the more addicted you are likely to be.

Calculate your nicotine dependence score using this calculator.[183]

Nicotine dependence calculator					score	
Number of cigarettes per day	1-4	5-15	16-25	>25		SCORING:
	0	1	2	3		0-3: low dependence
						4-6: high dependence
Time to first cigarette of the day (minutes)	>60	31-60	6-30	<5		
	0	1	2	3		
Total score					/6	

The 'strength' of the cigarettes you smoke is not a reliable guide to your nicotine needs when vaping. The reason is that smokers puff differently to get the right amount of nicotine they need. A smoker of light cigarettes could be puffing frequently and more intensely and still getting high levels of nicotine.

Measuring nicotine concentration

The concentration of nicotine is measured in two different ways. The most common method is in mg/mL (milligrams per millilitre). For example, a 6mg/mL e-juice has 6 milligrams of nicotine (by weight) in each millilitre (by volume). Often the 'per mL' (/mL) is dropped and it is expressed as 6mg. A 60mL bottle of 6mg/mL contains 360mg of nicotine.

Nicotine can also be measured as a percentage. A 5% nicotine e-liquid is made of 5 parts of nicotine and 95 parts of other liquids (PG, VG and flavourings) measured by volume.

A measurement in mg/mL can be converted to a percentage by dividing it by 10. So, a 6mg/mL e-liquid is the same strength as 0.6%.

Nicotine conversion table								
mg/mL	3	6	12	20	24	30	50	100
% nicotine by volume	0.3%	0.6%	1.2%	2%	2.4%	3%	5%	10%

Freebase nicotine or nicotine salt?

Nicotine liquid is available for vaping in two different forms: freebase nicotine and nicotine salt. Both are effective in replacing nicotine and equally potent, but there are important differences.

Freebase nicotine is mainly used in low concentrations in high wattage devices, such as box mods and vape pens. Freebase nicotine provides the familiar 'throat hit' (the sensation at the back of the throat) which is part of the smoking experience. At high concentrations, freebase nicotine can be harsh and irritating to the throat. Typical concentrations range from 3-24mg/mL (0.3-2.4%).

Nicotine salt is formed by adding an acid (such as benzoic, lactic or salicylic acid) to freebase nicotine. Nicotine salts are smoother to inhale and allow you to use higher doses with less throat irritation.[184] Nicotine salts are also absorbed more quickly than freebase nicotine and have a more rapid effect like nicotine from smoking. Nicotine salts do not give as strong a throat hit as smoking and may not be as satisfying for some smokers.

Nicotine salt is used in low-powered devices such as pod vapes and disposable vapes. These devices require a higher strength of nicotine to deliver an adequate dose but use lower volumes of liquid. Nicotine salts are used mostly in the 20-60mg/mL range (2-6%), however they can also be used in lower concentrations if preferred.

As a rough estimate, the throat hit of 6mg/mL freebase nicotine is similar to around 20mg/mL of nicotine salt.

What nicotine concentration should you start with?

When you first start to vape, it is best to get advice on the nicotine concentration from your doctor and the vape shop staff.

The starting nicotine level depends on how nicotine-dependent you are and the type of device you are using. Here are some guidelines for the nicotine concentration to start with for **mouth-to-lung** vaping.

Nicotine selection for mouth-to-lung vaping				
Device	Highly dependent heavy smoker		Low dependent light smoker	
	Concentration	Type of nicotine	Concentration	Type of nicotine
Cigalike	18-24mg/mL	freebase	6-18mg/mL	freebase
Disposable	50-60mg/mL	nicotine salt	25-30mg/mL	nicotine salt
Pre-filled pod vape	20-60mg/mL	nicotine salt	20-30mg/mL	nicotine salt
Re-fillable pod vape	20-30mg/mL	nicotine salt	20-25mg/mL	nicotine salt
	6-18mg/mL	freebase	6-9mg/mL	freebase
Vape pen	12-24mg/mL	freebase	3-12mg/mL	freebase
Box mod	6-18mg/mL	freebase	3-12mg/mL	freebase

Lower levels of nicotine are used for **direct-to-lung** (sub-ohm) vaping, usually 3-6mg/mL (0.3-0.6%) of freebase nicotine.

Most vapers start at a higher nicotine concentration to ensure they get enough nicotine when trying to quit smoking and then step down over time to lower levels.[171]

Propylene glycol (PG)

Propylene glycol (1,2-propanediol) is a clear, tasteless liquid found in almost all e-liquids. It is also used in a wide range of other products such as foods, medicines, cosmetics, asthma inhalers, air disinfectants and food flavourings. Another common use is for making theatre fog in stage productions.

Along with nicotine, PG helps to create the familiar throat hit which can help make the transition from smoking to vaping easier. PG also helps to carry the flavouring in the e-liquid. PG has antibacterial properties and may help to reduce infections.

PG is generally regarded as safe but there is limited experience with the effects of long-term inhalation. Some people can find it irritating in the mouth or lungs. A small number of people are allergic to PG and can use alternatives such as 1,3-propanediol.[185]

Vegetable glycerine (VG)

The other ingredient in almost all e-liquids is vegetable glycerine (VG), a clear, viscous, sweet tasting liquid. VG is also widely used in pharmaceuticals (such as cough syrups, creams), toothpaste and foods. It is generally regarded as very safe although there is limited information on the effects of long-term inhalation.

The main function of VG is to produce thicker, larger vape clouds with a smoother feel.

PG / VG ratio

E-liquids are made with different proportions of PG and VG, expressed as a PG / VG ratio, such as 50% PG / 50% VG, 70% PG / 30% VG, or 60% PG / 40% VG. Differing ratios of these two ingredients will alter the throat hit, strength of flavour and amount of cloud produced and are suitable for different devices.

E-liquids with higher PG levels are best suited to mouth-to-lung vaping with pod vapes and vape pens and give a stronger flavour and 'throat hit'. High PG liquids are thinner (less viscous) and are more prone to leaking from the device. They also deliver more nicotine than liquids with high VG levels.[186] People who are sensitive to PG, can reduce their PG level and increase the VG component.

E-liquids with higher VG levels are used more in direct-to-lung vaping. The greater the percentage of VG, the more vapour is produced. High VG liquids are thick and viscous and do not soak into coils as well. However, they are less likely to cause leakage.

Flavourings

Most smokers start vaping tobacco-flavoured e-liquid which more closely resembles the familiar taste of smoking. Over time, most progress to other flavours such as fruit, sweet, mint and food flavours, which don't remind you of smoking. A very small number of vapers use unflavoured e-liquids.

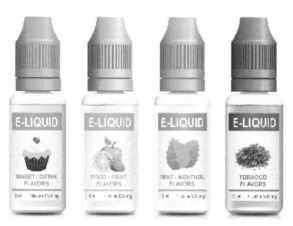

Popular e-liquid flavours

Flavours are an important part of vaping and make it more appealing as a replacement for smoking. Flavours have been shown to increase quit rates compared to non-flavoured e-liquids [187] and reduce the risk of returning to smoking.[188,189]

Certain flavouring chemicals are known to have potential risks and are best avoided. These include diacetyl (buttery),[190] cinnamaldehyde (cinnamon) [191] and benzaldehyde (cherry) [192] which are all banned in Australia.[118]

Small amounts of chemicals are produced when flavourings in e-liquid are heated. Although some of these chemicals are potentially harmful, they have so far not been associated with any serious risk.[84]

Most of the flavouring products are food flavourings and are safe to swallow, but less is known about their safety when inhaled. Some companies now conduct emission tests to identify the specific products in the vapour, and this is becoming more common.

So far, serious health effects from vaping flavours have been extremely rare. According to a recent report for the European Commission, 'To date, there is no specific data that specific flavourings used in the EU pose health risks for electronic cigarette users following repeated exposure.'[193] However, some flavours could potentially cause harm over time and this risk needs to be monitored.

Nevertheless, based on what we currently know about these chemicals they are certain to be much less harmful in the long term than continuing to smoke.

Pre-mixed or mix your own?

Your next decision is whether to buy ready-to-vape nicotine e-liquid or to mix your own.

Pre-mixed e-liquid

Most new vapers use pre-mixed, flavoured nicotine e-liquid, purchased in pre-filled pods or in a bottle for refilling their device. A wide range of nicotine concentrations and flavours are available in PG and VG. Commercial products are convenient, reasonably priced and generally prepared to a high standard. The most popular bottle sizes are 60mL and 100mL, but 30mL and 120mL bottles are also available.

Pre-mixed nicotine e-liquids can be purchased from international websites. They can also be purchased from selected Australian pharmacies if you have a prescription from a registered Australian medical practitioner who is an 'Authorised Prescriber' for nicotine.[38]

Nicotine shots and shortfills

Some pharmacies now sell 'nicotine shots' for mixing with 'shortfills'.

Nicotine shots are small bottles of freebase nicotine or nicotine salt (usually 10-20 mL) in various concentrations. The full bottle of nicotine is added to a 'shortfill' of your favourite flavoured e-liquid which can be purchased from a vape shop. Shortfill bottles have extra space to allow the nicotine shot to be added.

For example, adding a 10mL shot of 36mg/mL nicotine to a 60ml bottle (with 50mL of flavoured e-liquid) produces 60mL of 6mg/mL nicotine flavoured e-liquid.

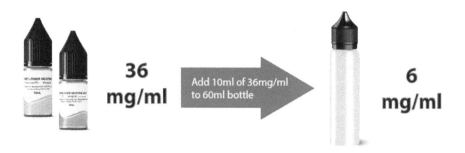

Adding a nicotine shot to a shortfill of flavoured e-liquid

Nicotine shots are safer for mixing than using 100mg/mL nicotine. They have child-resistant lids and require no measuring or syringes.

Nicotine shots and shortfills are popular in the UK and are now being used in Australia. The nicotine shots need a doctor's prescription in Australia.

Basic mixing

Basic mixing involves adding a small amount of highly concentrated nicotine (100mg/mL) to a bottle of nicotine-free e-juice (made of PG, VG and flavouring). High concentrations of nicotine should be handled carefully and stored safely.

You can use the chart below when using 100mg/mL nicotine liquid to prepare your preferred nicotine concentration in a particular bottle size. It can be used for freebase or nicotine salt liquids.

For example, to get a final nicotine concentration of 6mg/mL (0.6%) in a 60mL bottle, add 3.6 mL of 100mg/mL nicotine liquid to a 60ml bottle of flavoured e-liquid. Take out 3.6mL first so the final volume is 60mL. Ask the vape shop staff to help you do it the first time.

Nicotine mixing chart for unflavoured 100mg/mL nicotine

Bottle size	100ml	60ml	50ml	30ml
Final nicotine concentration (mg/mL)	Nicotine added (mL)	Nicotine added (mL)	Nicotine added (mL)	Nicotine added (mL)
1	1	0.6	0.5	0.3
2	2	1.2	1	0.6
3	3	1.8	1.5	0.9
4	4	2.4	2	1.2
5	5	3	2.5	1.5
6	6	3.6	3	1.8
9	9	5.4	4.5	2.7
12	12	7.2	6	3.6
15	15	9	7.5	4.5
18	18	10.8	9	5.4
25	25	15	12.5	7.5
35	35	21	17.5	10.5
50	50	30	50	15

Advanced DIY (do-it-yourself) mixing

More advanced DIY mixing involves following a 'recipe' or your own formula and measuring and mixing the individual ingredients of the e-liquid.

For mixing you need high concentrations of nicotine liquid, usually 100mg/mL. If your doctor thinks this is appropriate to help you quit smoking, this can be prescribed and three months' supply at a time can be imported under the TGA Personal Importation Scheme or purchased from a participating pharmacy.[36]

DIY mixing is considerably cheaper than using commercial pre-mixed juices and allows you to customise your e-liquid to your needs.

The steps involved in DIY mixing are:

1. Find or create a recipe. Numerous free tested recipes are available online, for example from www.e-liquid-recipes.com or https://alltheflavors.com/recipes, or you can make up your own.

2. Buy your ingredients and other supplies from an online vendor, local vape shop or a participating Australian pharmacy.

Ingredients to buy

- Propylene glycol and vegetable glycerine. These can be purchased individually or pre-mixed in your preferred ratio, e.g. 50% PG / 50% VG or 75% PG / 25% VG. Liquids should be pharmaceutical grade or USP quality (United States Pharmacopoeia) to reduce the risk of impurities.

- Concentrated (100mg/mL) pharmaceutical grade nicotine liquid, which is usually supplied in PG. Pure nicotine (almost 1,000mg/mL) is far too strong and toxic and should never be used for mixing.

- Flavour concentrates. Only use concentrates made specifically for vaping and avoid any oil-based liquids. You can use one flavour or create your own taste sensation with a combination!

Other supplies

These are available as a DIY kit or you can buy the items individually from vape shops or pharmacies:

- Plastic child-resistant dropper bottles for storing your creations
- Syringes of various sizes, blunt dispensing needles, and droppers

- Labels

- Disposable gloves and goggles to protect your eyes in case splashes occur when mixing

- An electronic scale with 0.01-gram precision if mixing by weight

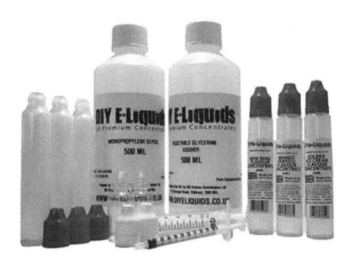

Commercial DIY mixing kit

3. Unless you are a maths genius, it is best to use an online calculator to work out what volume or weight of each ingredient to add to your mixture. Many free 'online-ready' calculators are available, for example at www.e-liquid-recipes.com or https://alltheflavors.com/recipes, or you can download one from http://www.ejuice.breaktru.com. Simply enter into the calculator the nicotine concentration you want, the desired PG / VG ratio and the percentage of flavours as shown in your recipe.

4. Measure the individual ingredients with a syringe and blunt needle or pipette and mix them together in a labelled plastic bottle with a child-resistant lid. An alternative method is to weigh ingredients using an electronic scale. Store the final product in a child-safe place.

5. 'Steeping'. Some e-liquids need time to blend and settle after mixing for best results and this can take days or weeks. Most recipes come with a recommended steeping time.

Safety

Mixing your own e-liquids is inherently riskier than purchasing products. Great care should be taken in handling concentrated nicotine, accurately measuring ingredients and avoiding exposure to children and pets.

Like all household chemicals, nicotine e-liquids should be stored safely out of the reach of children and pets and kept in unbreakable bottles with childproof lids. Never store nicotine liquid in unlabelled or drink containers. Concentrated nicotine is best stored in a freezer in a locked bag.

Mixing should never be done while young children are around as it only takes a moment of inattention for accidents to occur.

It is good practice to wear gloves and consider goggles when using highly concentrated nicotine solutions. Spills should be promptly cleaned up and nicotine liquid washed from the skin.

Resources

If you are considering mixing your own e-liquids, it is important to do some research. Speak to your local vape shop staff or other experienced mixers, read online resources or ask questions on a DIY vaping forum.

DIY Downunder 18+ is an excellent Facebook group for Australian vapers who mix their own e-liquids. New users are welcome to join and get advice from experienced mixers: https://www.facebook.com/groups/diydownunder.

Other good resources are the DIY subreddit, https://www.reddit.com/r/DIY_eJuice, this DIY forum https://forum.e-liquid-recipes.com and a free guide to 'Mastering the Art of DIY Vapor' here https://bit.ly/3stkmTH.

Samantha and her mother

Samantha and her mother have bipolar disorder.   Both quit smoking by switching to vaping.

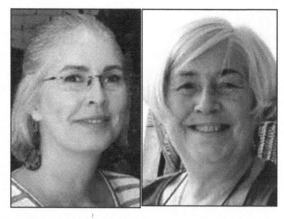

Samantha writes, 'I tried my first cigarette at eleven years of age and became a habitual smoker by my mid-twenties.'

I enjoyed smoking but desperately wanted to quit. I tried 'cold turkey' many times, nicotine patches and hypnosis, all without success. I read Allen Carr's book on stopping smoking which also did not work.

All up, I smoked daily for fifteen years, only quitting when I fell pregnant, but started again when my son was a few months old.

Almost seven years ago, a friend introduced me to vaping and I finally found something that worked. After about four months of vaping and smoking together, I quit cigarettes completely.

After a few weeks, my post-nasal drip at night disappeared and my chest no longer wheezed in the morning. I can exercise five days a week and feel great. My relationship with my husband has improved enormously. I am no longer subjecting my son to the smell of smoking (I always smoked outside) and I am a better role model for him.

I never thought I would be able to stop smoking cigarettes, I enjoyed them and became anxious at each quit attempt. I am so grateful for the invention of nicotine vaping which allows me to enjoy nicotine in a significantly less harmful way.

I introduced my mother to vaping and she was also able to quit cigarettes and loves vaping. My mother and I both have bipolar disorder and find nicotine particularly useful in managing stress. In addition to improving my health, I have also saved a huge amount of money by switching from cigarettes to vaping. I use a compact box mod with 15-18mg/mL nicotine (mouth-to-lung). I now mix my own e-liquids and enjoy the DIY hobby side of vaping which also saves money.

I have no current plans to quit vaping but realise it may become even more difficult due to the Australian government's hard-line prescription model. I would unreservedly recommend vaping over smoking, but the new laws due to come into effect from October 2021 will make it very difficult for a hardened smoker to switch.

11

VISIT YOUR GP

Take-home messages

- It is legal to vape nicotine in Australia if you have a nicotine prescription
- If you need nicotine e-liquid, see your GP to discuss getting a prescription
- Your doctor will assess whether vaping nicotine is appropriate for you
- Nicotine e-liquid can be imported from overseas, or purchased from selected Australian pharmacies
- Your GP may provide other counselling and support to help you quit
- If your GP is not able to assist, you can get a second opinion

In Australia, once you have chosen a vaporiser and e-liquid, the next step is to visit your GP to discuss getting a nicotine prescription and support for your quit attempt. As discussed on page 62, you need to have a prescription from a registered Australian doctor to legally import, possess or use nicotine liquid in Australia. Before writing a prescription, your doctor needs to decide if the product is appropriate for you.

The peak Australian GP body, the Royal Australian College of General Practitioners recognises a role for vaping as a second-line treatment for smokers who are otherwise unable to quit with other methods. The 2021 guidelines state:

'For people who have tried to achieve smoking cessation with first-line therapy (combination of behavioural support and TGA-approved pharmacotherapy) but failed and are still motivated to quit smoking, NVPs [Nicotine Vaping Products] may be a reasonable intervention to recommend along with behavioural support.'[4]

GPs are advised to discuss with patients that

- Due to the lack of available evidence, the long-term health effects of nicotine vaping products are unknown.
- Nicotine vaping products are not registered therapeutic goods in Australia and therefore their safety, efficacy and quality have not been established.
- There is a lack of uniformity in vaping devices and nicotine vaping products, which increases the uncertainties associated with their use.
- To maximise possible benefit and minimise risk of harms, dual use (smoking and vaping) should be avoided and long-term use should be minimised.
- It is important for the patient to return for regular review and monitoring

Visiting your GP

GPs are well-qualified to help you quit smoking and their advice and support can increase your chance of success. Your doctor can discuss first-line quitting aids such as nicotine replacement therapy, varenicline (Champix) and bupropion (Zyban) along with behavioural counselling.

If these have not worked or are not suitable, vaping nicotine may be a good choice.

At the consultation, tell your doctor about your past attempts to quit and why you would like to try vaping nicotine. If your doctor supports the decision you will need to discuss:

- Whether you would like to import e-liquid or buy it from a pharmacy. All GPs can legally write a nicotine prescription for importing nicotine liquid from overseas. However, if you want to purchase nicotine from an Australian chemist shop or online pharmacy, your doctor needs to register to be an 'Authorised Prescriber' of nicotine prior to your visit.[38] Some doctors may not wish to register for this scheme.

- Your starting nicotine concentration. This is based on how dependent on nicotine you are and what device you will be using. Discuss this with the vape shop staff and your GP.

- If importing nicotine e-liquid, how much you will need for a three-month period. The average volume used for mouth-to-lung vaping is 2-5mL per day, or up to 450mL for three months, although some vapers use a lot more. With pre-filled pod vapes, you will need ninety pods every three months if using one daily.

Advice given to GPs

The latest RACGP guidelines provide the following advice to GPs:[4]

1. Recommend new vapers use 'closed' systems (with pre-filled pods or cartridges) and avoid 'open' (refillable) systems to minimise risk. Advise current users of open systems to change to nicotine freebase concentrations of ≤20mg/mL and/or to a closed system.

2. Do not recommend disposables due to waste and unspecified safety issues, particularly those with nicotine salts >20mg/mL.

3. Write nicotine prescriptions for Australian pharmacies instead of for importation from overseas suppliers under the Personal Importation Scheme.

4. Avoid freebase nicotine over 20mg/mL.

5. Do not prescribe nicotine e-liquid concentrations of 100mg/mL and discourage DIY mixing.

6. Limit each prescription to a maximum of 3 months.

7. Where possible, avoid flavours or limit to tobacco flavour.

8. Provide follow-up and behavioural support.

What if my GP won't prescribe nicotine?

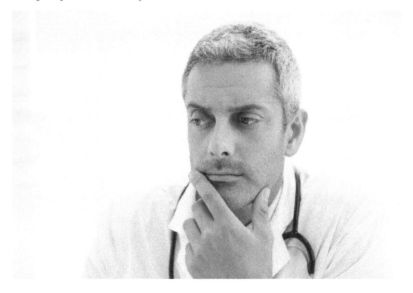

Most GPs have received little or no training about vaping

Don't be discouraged if your GP is not able to help. Most GPs have received very little or no education on vaping nicotine. Furthermore, doctors have been discouraged from prescribing nicotine by the Australian Medical Association and other medical bodies and most do not have the time to research the evidence themselves. You may wish to get an opinion from another doctor.

If your GP is not supportive, avoid getting angry. Politely and respect-fully point out that you have researched the area and know that vaping is a lot less risky than smoking and is a more effective quitting method than nicotine replacement therapy.

There are two lists of Australian GPs who are available to discuss whether vaping is suitable for you. These doctors have an interest in smoking, are well informed about vaping and can provide a prescription if it is appropriate. They are available from:

1. The Australian Tobacco Harm Reduction Association, www.athra.org.au/doctors

2. The Therapeutic Goods Administration, https://www.tga.gov.au/authorised-prescribers-unapproved-nicotine-vaping-products

Quitting support from your GP

Support from your GP can help you quit smoking whether you are using conventional quit smoking medication or vaping nicotine. This help could include:

- Other quitting methods which may be suitable for you. Have you used them correctly? Are there other methods you could try?

- Assessing whether you are dependent on nicotine.

- Helping manage your barriers to quitting, such as weight gain and stress.

- Coping strategies. Cravings for a cigarette are often triggered by specific situations, people, or moods. Your GP can help you identify triggers or cues and help you plan coping strategies for when they occur after quitting.

- Lifestyle changes. You are more likely to quit smoking if you can make other healthy lifestyle changes at the same time. Exercise is recommended for all smokers trying to quit. Exercise reduces cravings and stress, reduces weight gain, helps prevent relapse and has many other health benefits. Consider a new hobby or sport to fill the extra time you will have after quitting. Consider other changes such as healthier eating.

- Caffeine. When smokers drink coffee, caffeine is eliminated from the body more quickly than by non-smokers. After quitting, caffeine levels rise and you can develop 'caffeine toxicity', which can cause agitation, headaches and insomnia. Reducing caffeine by half is recommended when you quit.

- Alcohol often triggers a strong urge to smoke and the more you drink the more likely you are to relapse to smoking. It is a good idea to avoid alcohol for the first two to three weeks if possible and reduce your alcohol intake after that if necessary.

- Other strategies such as getting support from family and friends and setting yourself some well-earned rewards for staying quit, such as a massage, a session with a personal trainer or a holiday.

- Drug interactions with smoking. When you stop smoking (even if you switch to vaping) the dose of certain drugs may need to be reduced. This is especially important for clozapine and olanzapine (anti-psychotics), fluvoxamine (an antidepressant) and warfarin (blood thinner) but smoking can also affect other drugs. Speak to your GP when you switch if you are taking medications.

- Your GP may recommend a quit smoking app for your smartphone, such as Smoke Free (smoke-freeapp.com), a free, popular vape-friendly stop smoking app. In the last twelve months, over 66,500 Australia smokers downloaded it to help them stop smoking. My QuitBuddy is also popular.

- Seeing your doctor for further visits after quitting can be very helpful.

GP training on nicotine and vaping

GPs can log into the Health Professionals section of the ATHRA website (www.athra.org.au) for more information about vaping. Information is available on:

- The safety and effectiveness of vaping
- The legality of vaping and prescribing nicotine
- How to write a nicotine prescription
- How to counsel patients about vaping
- Further handouts, references and reports on vaping

Dr Kevin Murphy

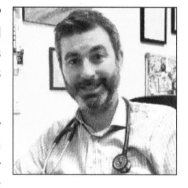

Kevin is an Adelaide-based GP who quit smoking with vaping and subsequently stopped vaping as well. Now he wants to help others do the same thing. This is his story.

'I grew up in Ireland and everybody in my family smoked. I took it up in my mid-teens and became heavily addicted very quickly. Over the next fifteen years or so, I made multiple unfruitful attempts to quit. I used all the available medicines at one time or another: nicotine replacement therapy, bupropion and varenicline.

I had resigned myself to a lifetime of being a 'tobacco slave'. Then I learned about vaping, so decided to try it in 2012, starting with a cigalike.

I never smoked another cigarette after I took up vaping. It ticked all of the boxes for me: it delivered the nicotine, it gave me that 'throat hit', it occupied my hands, as well as being far, far less harmful to my health than tobacco.

Immediately on switching from tobacco to vaping I felt my health improve. The beginnings of a smokers' cough vanished, I had more energy and started to exercise (whilst not being limited by shortness of breath). The horrible smell disappeared and my self-esteem improved.

I graduated to a box mod with pre-mixed 18mg/mL nicotine e-liquid and finally ceased vaping at the end of 2019 after gradually reducing nicotine levels to 2mg/mL then quitting. I fervently believe that if I had not switched to vaping, I would still be using tobacco.

Speaking as a doctor who has appraised the available evidence, and as an ex-smoker and ex-vaper, there is absolutely, unequivocally no doubt in my mind that switching from smoking to vaping nicotine is a no-brainer.

Advising smokers about vaping as a far safer alternative to combustible cigarettes is something that makes plain common sense to me, and all doctors across the board should be doing it. The fact that this isn't yet happening is of deep concern to me.'

12

WHERE TO BUY VAPING PRODUCTS

Take-home messages

- Buy your vaping devices, pods, coils, accessories and nicotine-free e-liquids from your local vape shop
- Vape shops provide expert support and advice
- Nicotine e-liquid can be purchased from overseas websites or from selected Australian pharmacies
- The purchase of black-market e-liquid is very risky and is not recommended

Brick-and-mortar vape shops

In a vape shop, you can see and handle different vaping devices and get expert advice from experienced vapers. Staff can help you select a device and show you how to operate, fill, maintain and use it safely. Vape shops also sell accessories such as replacement coils, spare pods and batteries.

Australian vape shops are not allowed by law to sell nicotine liquid but can sell nicotine-free juice. Most vape shops allow you to sample ('taste') different flavours in-store before you buy. Many vapers purchase these liquids and mix them with unflavoured concentrated nicotine (100mg/mL) or 'nicotine shots' imported from overseas or purchased from participating Australian pharmacies with a prescription.

Most beginners purchase pre-mixed, flavoured nicotine e-liquid from overseas websites or participating pharmacies.

The display and sale of vaping products is strictly regulated by state and territory laws. For example, in NSW, vaping products cannot be displayed in-store except when requested by a customer. Shops are also required to block windows so that vaping products cannot be seen by the public from outside the premises, making it harder for customers to locate stores. Sales can only be made from one register in each store.[194]

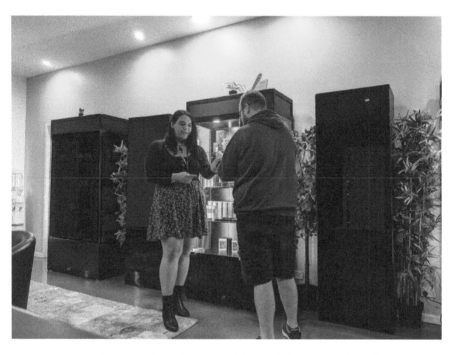

A vape shop in Sydney showing cabinets with concealed products

In Western Australia, it is illegal to sell a complete vaping device. However, vape shops sell individual parts which can be assembled.

Vape shops are mostly located in major urban areas, but increasingly shops are opening in rural and regional locations. Some brands have several outlets and larger chains are also starting to appear. See the table below to find a vape shop near you.

Finding a vape shop near you

www.aussievapedirectory.com lists 152 Australian stores.

www.vapetrotter.com lists 26,000 retail stores globally, including 160 in Australia.

Australian websites

Most Australian brick-and-mortar vape stores also have an online presence to sell their products. Some Australian vape suppliers are online only. Australian websites are not allowed to sell nicotine liquid, even if you have a prescription.

In South Australia, the online sale of all vaping products is banned. It is illegal for local, interstate and international businesses to sell any vaping supplies to residents of the state. South Australian residents can still purchase supplies from local brick-and-mortar vape shops.

Vapem8

Vapem8 is an Australian price comparison website for all vaping products. If you are looking for a particular device or e-liquid you can compare the prices from a wide range of vendors. Go to www.vapem8.com.au.

International websites

You can import three months' supply of nicotine at a time for personal use to quit smoking under the Therapeutic Goods Administration Personal Importation Scheme with a prescription from an Australian doctor.[36] Most users purchase their nicotine liquid from New Zealand suppliers who can usually arrange delivery in two to three days. Others import from the UK or China, but the buyer should always beware. You can find out which suppliers are reputable and popular from vape forums or vape shop staff.

Ordering from the US has become more difficult since March 2021 due to changes in the PACT Act (Prevent All Cigarette Trafficking Act).[195]

Onerous restrictions on shipping vape products have been introduced and most courier companies no longer make deliveries to Australia.

You should upload or email a copy of your prescription to the vendor so it can be enclosed with your order.[196] Australian Border Force (ABF) officials may stop the parcel at the border. If there is no prescription enclosed the ABF can destroy the goods and you may also face penalties for importing a prohibited substance. The current penalty is up to $222,000 for each offence.[197]

Australian pharmacies

Nicotine e-liquid can also be purchased from a small number of Australian (physical or online) pharmacies if you have a prescription under the 'Authorised Prescriber Scheme'.[38] Only doctors who have applied to the Therapeutic Goods Administration to become Authorised Prescribers for nicotine e-liquid can write scripts for this purpose. Check if your doctor is an Authorised Prescriber. A list of Authorised Prescribers who give permission to be listed publicly is available at https://www.tga.gov.au/authorised-prescribers-unapproved-nicotine-vaping-products.

Pharmacies can supply imported commercial products or can make (compound) them from the basic ingredients.

1. Imported e-liquids

Australian pharmacies can sell commercial nicotine e-liquid sourced from overseas. However, there are thousands of pods, e-liquid brands and flavours currently on the market and only a small fraction of these will be available.

Check with the pharmacy if the product you want is available and how long it will take to get it.

2. Compounding pharmacies

Registered compounding pharmacies can prepare customised nicotine e-liquid made from the individual ingredients when provided with a prescription from an Authorised Prescriber. Ask the compounding pharmacy if they prepare nicotine e-liquids and what flavours are available. Compounded preparations can be made with different nicotine concentrations, PG / VG ratios and in a range of flavours.

Other retail outlets

No Australian retail outlets other than pharmacies can legally sell nicotine e-liquid.

Non-nicotine e-liquids and vaping devices are also available from some tobacconists and general stores. These outlets offer a smaller range of products and staff may not be able to provide the same level of advice and support found in vape shops.

Traveller's exemption

The traveller's exemption allows people entering Australia from over-seas to carry their vaping device and nicotine e-liquid with them for their own personal use.[198]

You can bring up to three months' supply of nicotine e-liquid at a time if you have a prescription from an Australian doctor. Keep the original packaging intact so it can be easily identified.[198]

Black-market nicotine

It is illegal to sell liquid nicotine in Australia (except from pharmacies) but a thriving black-market is the inevitable result of Australia's strict regulation. Purchase of illegal nicotine 'under-the-counter' is strongly discouraged. There are no guarantees of product quality or safety or that the liquid is what it claims to be.

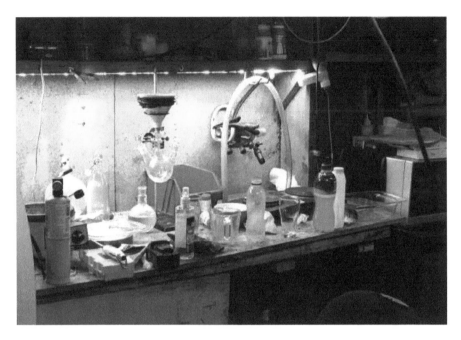

An illicit drug laboratory

Mal

Mal smoked for 40 years and finally quit with vaping. He has now established a vape business to help other smokers quit.

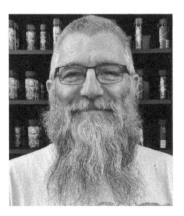

'After my mother died of lung cancer in early 2000, I tried everything to stop smoking, including nicotine patches, gum, lozenges, sprays, acupuncture and hypnotherapy. A short trial with Champix sent me to the 'dark side' and was terrifying.

After everything failed, I resigned myself to an early death from smoking, just like my mother.

Then, seven years ago I discovered vaping, and quit smoking overnight!

Over the following weeks I noticed exciting changes. Bland food tasted better — I guess my taste buds were reawakening. I started to smell things again. My doctor confirmed that my asthma was improving, and the early signs of emphysema were receding.

Over the next year I helped many friends to also make the change. All my smoking friends asked what I was doing. What was the device I was 'smoking'? Can I try it? Can I get them one? I started to order a few vaporisers for friends from China. The success rate for my friends was nearly 100%.

I started selling vape pens and liquids from under a gazebo at a local café on weekends, then moved to Parklea Markets in early 2015. A few months later I quit my corporate job to open a vape shop and help many more people quit tobacco.

Owning a vape shop has been the most rewarding time of my life. I love seeing the amazement when a new customer tries a vape for the first time. I love seeing new vapers return after a few days, sharing their excitement about quitting cigarettes. I love to hear of the physical transformations they go through, just as I had. I love helping people to quit tobacco.

I only wish vaping was around earlier for my mother.'

Mal is the managing director of Vapour Power, www.vapourpower. com.au

13

START VAPING

Take-home messages

- Take slow three to four second puffs whenever you get the urge to smoke
- It takes some people a while to adjust to vaping but it becomes more satisfying with practice
- It is safe to vape and smoke for a while, until you are ready to let go of the ciggies
- Don't be afraid to increase the nicotine concentration if needed
- Make sure you vape frequently enough to satisfy your cravings
- Drink more water to prevent a dry mouth
- Keep trying until you find the combination of device, nicotine concentration and flavour that works for you
- Vape courteously when around others as you do when smoking
- Always keep spare coils, adequate e-liquid supplies and a spare charged device available
- It is very important to stop smoking completely
- Once you have quit smoking, stop vaping if you can, but continue long-term if vaping is keeping you from relapsing to smoking

Now that you have a vaping device, e-liquid and spare coils or pods, it's time to get started!

Some people find vaping immediately satisfying while others take longer to adjust. There is no right or wrong timeframe and no need to rush.

Most vapers say that vaping becomes more satisfying with practice. Over time you learn to fine-tune your puffing technique and get more nicotine from each puff.[199] It may take some months or even a year or two before you are ready to completely let go of your old friend, cigarettes. It is quite safe to vape and smoke together for a while (known as 'dual use') until you are ready to stop smoking for good.

If other people say you are still smoking, you can assure them that this is not the case. There is no smoke in a vape, so none of the harmful tar, carbon monoxide and other toxins that you get from a smoked cigarette.

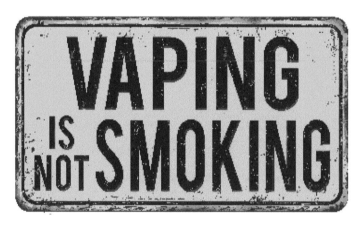

Tell people that you are vaping to quit smoking. That will help to stop them offering you cigarettes and might even encourage them to try vaping as well.

How to puff

Using a vape is a little different to smoking. Experienced vapers take longer puffs, about three to four seconds compared to a typical puff on a cigarette of about one to two seconds.[200,201]This is because the coil only heats up when you are inhaling. Longer puffs keep the coil heated for longer, releasing more vapour and nicotine. If you are not getting enough nicotine, you can also take more frequent puffs.

Inhaling faster does not increase nicotine intake but can cause unpleasant throat irritation.

As described earlier (page 77), there are two ways of inhaling. Most newbie vapers prefer mouth-to-lung vaping (MTL) which is more similar to smoking. MTL vaping is a two-step process. First, draw the vapour into the mouth, then inhale it into the lungs as a second step.

When you first start vaping, take several small puffs to see how it feels. Coughing is common in the early stages, but almost always resolves over the first week. Remember that it takes a little longer to feel the effects of nicotine compared to smoking.

Later, you may wish to try direct-to-lung vaping (DTL) which involves drawing the vapour directly into your lungs. This is a very different technique to smoking and generally requires a different type of vaping device or coil. Very few vapers start with DTL vaping.

When to vape

Use your vape when you get the urge to smoke.

Some vapers 'graze' throughout the day, having a puff or a few puffs when needed.[201] This is different to smoking, where you need to finish the whole cigarette. Other vapers prefer a discrete vaping break, having ten to twelve puffs as you would with a cigarette break.

Make sure you vape every day if you want to quit. Research has shown that daily use is far more effective for quitting smoking than vaping less frequently.[153]

Make sure you get enough nicotine

Chapter 10 explains how to select your starting nicotine concentration based on your nicotine dependence and the vaping device you are using.

One of the most common reasons for a failed vaping attempt is not getting enough nicotine due to falsely believing that nicotine causes significant harm. In fact, almost all the harm from smoking is caused by over 7,000 chemicals in smoke created by burning tobacco, not nicotine.[11]

You should get as much nicotine as you need to satisfy your cravings. Generally, regular vapers get the same amount of nicotine from vaping as they did from smoking.[186] If you are not getting enough nicotine you will try to get it from cigarettes. You can increase your nicotine intake in several ways:

1. Increase the nicotine concentration of your e-liquid. Don't be afraid of nicotine. It has minor harmful effects in the doses used in vaping. If an increase in freebase nicotine is too harsh on the throat, switch to nicotine salt. Nicotine salt is smoother and better tolerated.

2. Have longer puffs (at least three to four seconds) and puff more frequently during the day. Don't be afraid to vape as often as you need. It can help to work out how many puffs a day you took while smoking and make sure you are puffing on your vape at least as often.

3. You can use more nicotine at certain times of the day when cravings are stronger, such as in the morning on waking or when stressed. It can be useful to keep two devices or pods on the go – one with higher nicotine e-liquid for when you really need to manage the urge for a cigarette, the other with less nicotine for when you just want to puff.

4. Using a nicotine patch while vaping nicotine can increase quit rates.[144] The nicotine patch works in the background throughout the day and vaping helps you cope with the regular smoking triggers such as coffee or stress. Discuss this with your doctor if needed.

5. Use a more powerful device. More powerful devices and lower resistance coils release more nicotine.

Be persistent

If you are not finding vaping nicotine satisfying immediately, don't give up! There is a learning curve with vaping and sometimes a prolonged adjustment period.[171] The advice from experienced vapers is to experiment with different nicotine concentrations, device types and flavours until you find the right combination that works for you.[172] For example, if a pod vape is not working for you, try a vape pen or mod. Get advice from your local vape shop, an online forum, or other vapers if you are unsure how to proceed.

Over time, vaping becomes more rewarding. Vapers automatically adjust their puffing technique by taking fewer and longer puffs which are more effective.[199] Over the first four weeks, you learn to increase your nicotine intake to get the effect you need.[202]

Be prepared

When you smoked, it was easy to buy another packet of cigarettes or a lighter if you ran out. It's not so easy with vaping supplies in Australia and you need a backup plan.

Once you have found a model that suits you, purchase a second device or a spare battery (if using removable batteries) and keep it charged. Many vapers have relapsed to smoking when their vape has been lost, broken or run flat.

Don't forget that it may take a few days to get more e-liquid delivered from your favourite overseas supplier or pharmacy. Plan ahead and make sure to have enough juice to keep you going.

Make sure you take your vape with you when you leave home and always have spare coils and extra e-liquid in case you need them.

Side-effects

The most common side-effects from vaping (and smoking) are throat or mouth irritation, headache, cough and nausea. These reactions are usually mild and tend to settle over time.[9]

You are likely to find that your mouth feels quite dry during the first few days – drinking extra sips of water will help manage this.

It is almost impossible to harm yourself by overdosing when vaping nicotine. If you are getting too much nicotine, you may experience nausea, light-headedness or palpitations. If this occurs, have a break and puff less frequently or have shorter puffs and it will quickly pass. Better still, try to reduce the number of cigarettes you are smoking to reduce your nicotine intake.

Serious side-effects from vaping are extremely rare.

Your nicotine prescription

When ordering nicotine liquid from overseas, send a copy of the prescription to the retailer so it can be returned with your order. This will avoid a delay in receiving your goods.

If you have ordered a quantity of nicotine or a concentration that is greater than what is specified on your prescription, the order may not be released by the Border Force and is likely to be destroyed.

Keep an image of your nicotine script on your smartphone in case it is required by authorities. It is a criminal offence to possess nicotine in Australia without one.

Vaping etiquette

Good vaping etiquette is simply good manners and helps to build community support for vaping. Second-hand vapour has not been shown to have harmful effects on people around you. However other people have a right to fresh air.

Courteous vaping means following the social guidelines you use when smoking. These include:

- Try to avoid vaping around other people or only exhale small clouds when this is not possible. It is also good manners to ask people around you before you start vaping.

- Try not to vape around children, pregnant women or people with heart or lung conditions.
- Avoid vaping in confined spaces or where people are eating.
- Use the vaping or smoking area if one is provided.
- Ask your host's permission before vaping in their home.

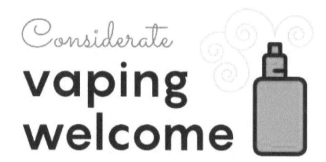

Sign by New Nicotine Alliance in the United Kingdom

Flavours

Most smokers who switch to vaping start with tobacco-flavoured e-liquid. This is the taste they are familiar with and research shows it eases the transition away from smoking. However, tobacco-flavouring is artificially made and does not taste exactly like the burning tobacco leaf you are used to. There are many different tobacco flavoured e-liquids and some will suit you better than others.

Once you are an established vaper, don't be afraid to explore the many fruit, sweet, mint and beverage flavours available which make vaping more enjoyable. Most vapers say these non-tobacco flavours help to break the association with tobacco smoking.

Changing flavours in a cigalike or pod device is easy – you just swap the cartridge or pod. In a tank model, you need to remove the tank, drain the e-liquid and take out the coil. E-liquids are not oils, but are water soluble, so you can rinse the tank with hot water and soap as well if needed and let the tank air-dry. Then re-insert the coil and refill the tank with the new flavoured e-liquid. You can re-use the old coil, but your first few hits will be a mixture of both flavours.

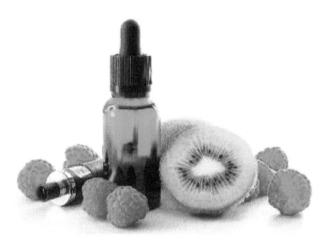

Fruit flavours are most popular

Stealth vaping

There may be times when you are allowed to vape but want to avoid drawing attention to yourself. Stealth vaping is a way to vape with small or almost invisible clouds.

The best devices for stealth vaping are low-powered, compact pod devices with a high resistance coil. E-liquids with a higher PG /VG ratio (i.e. more PG) are best as they produce less vapour.

To stealth vape, take short puffs and try to delay the exhale for a little longer than usual. It can be more effective to take a breath, remove the vape from your mouth, then inhale air and hold your breath before you breathe out.

When you exhale, purse your lips and blow a fine stream of vapour downward and away from any onlookers or into your hand. You can also exhale into a handkerchief or scarf to reduce visible clouds.

If the device has an LED light at the tip, make sure to cover it when you inhale.

When to stop smoking

You will get the greatest health benefits when you stop smoking completely. Even one cigarette a day is very harmful.

Some smokers who start vaping cease smoking immediately. Others continue to smoke and vape for a while until they are ready to quit cigarettes. This can take months, or even a year or two.[182]

Try to gradually reduce the number of cigarettes you smoke over time and replace them with vaping. Some people find a reduction schedule helpful. Others prefer to set a quit day.

Another strategy is to stop smoking completely for the first three days and vape as much as you need. This works very well for some smokers.

Some people have a hard time giving up certain cigarettes each day, such as on waking or when stressed. Vaping may not seem as satisfying as smoking at these times, but to fully quit smoking you need to switch to vaping even at these times. It may not seem as satisfying at first, but it will become easier over time. Using higher nicotine concentrations at these times can help.

If you are finding it difficult to stop smoking you may need a higher concentration of nicotine, more frequent puffing or a different vaping device. Get some advice from a vaping forum or the staff at your local vape shop.

Once you have quit, get rid of those cigarettes! Don't leave them lying around as the temptation may be too much at certain times. Most ex-smokers know that having 'just one' is usually the beginning of going back to smoking.

When to stop vaping

It is always best for your health to quit vaping if you can. Long-term vaping carries some risk and there may be future harms we don't yet know about. Quitting vaping will also save you money and finally give you freedom from nicotine!

Aim to quit vaping when you feel sure you won't go back to smoking. Some people stop vaping within three to six months, others continue much longer because they enjoy vaping and find it keeps them from smoking. Continuing to vape is always safer than relapsing to smoking.

To stop vaping you can gradually vape less often or use lower nicotine concentrations over time, for example going from 12mg/mL to 6mg/mL to 3mg/mL. You may find that vaping nicotine-free liquid is effective. If you are more dependent on nicotine you may find that temporarily adding nicotine patch or gum makes the transition easier. It is best to discuss this with your doctor.

You can also set rules for yourself about where and when you vape, gradually reducing your usage. Try to avoid situations where you are most likely to vape for a while, such as having a drink with friends.

If you find you are compensating by vaping more often or inhaling more deeply when cutting down you may not be ready to stop vaping yet.

After you have quit smoking and vaping, it is a good idea to keep your vape handy. If you are about to undo all that hard work that you put into quitting, use the vape instead. It will keep you smoke-free. If you don't want to vape again, you could use nicotine gum or lozenges to help at difficult times.

However, if you do have a slip, don't feel bad and beat yourself up. It happens. Get back on the vaping and commit to quitting right away.

Spread the word

Now that vaping has helped you finally quit smoking, it's time to tell your friends, family, doctor and workmates who still smoke. Tell them how much better you feel and how much money you have saved.

Also tell your local members of parliament. Ring them or write a short, polite letter and ask for a brief meeting to explain how vaping has helped you. Write to your local newspaper, ring talkback radio and spread the word!

Kelli

Kelli is a thirty-one-year-old mother of three children from Kempsey, New South Wales. She says that vaping 'has honestly, whole-heartedly saved my life.'

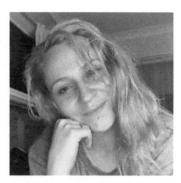

Kelli started smoking at the age of eleven to help her cope with a difficult upbringing. Self-medicating with nicotine and other substances made life bearable and helped her focus but led to a life-long battle with addiction. She fell pregnant at sixteen and desperately tried to quit but couldn't.

But she kept trying. 'Champix resulted in me becoming violent, agitated and almost like I was living in a nightmare. I still smoked during Champix and patch use. I tried inhalers, and that awful gum that burnt and left ulcers. Patches either made me feel so nauseous I'd rip them off and go back to smoking or had no effect and I still smoked while having them on.'

Eventually, her mum encouraged her to try vaping, something she had been doing herself for a few months. The mechanical action of hand-to-mouth, inhale, exhale, were still there but she was still craving cigarettes and other stimulants. 'Then I started using nicotine and I stopped smoking. That is what I needed and it was instant.'

'Nicotine helped settle my ADHD. It calmed me in a way that ADHD medications never did, making me less fidgety and able to control myself. My asthma totally cleared for the first time in years. I have no more morning cough or wheeze and no longer take asthma medication.'

'Within four or so months, life was as close to normal as I could ever have imagined it! For the first time ever since a kid I didn't feel sick!'

'When vaping nicotine, I also noticed the need for other substances declined. I have something now, that allows me to live a life, without multiple drugs, without risk of relapse, without major risks to myself or others.'

'I have now been vaping for four years. It has honestly, whole-heartedly, saved my life, my physical self, and who I am.'

You can't ask for more than that!

14

VAPE SAFELY

Take-home messages

- Always keep nicotine in child-resistant containers out of the reach of children and pets, preferably in a locked cupboard

- Use disposable gloves when handling nicotine, especially concentrated liquids

- Only buy e-liquid from reputable sellers

- Charge your device with the USB cable supplied, in a computer, TV or game console

- Only use low-amp wall charging adapters (0.5-1 amp) if using mains power

- Do not leave batteries unattended while charging and unplug when charged

- Charge removable batteries in an external battery charger on a non-flammable surface

- Never carry loose batteries in your pocket or purse without a plastic case

No vaping products have been approved by Australia's medicines regulator, the Therapeutic Goods Administration. However, modern devices are continuing to improve in quality and safety. The risk of harm from modern regulated devices from reputable manufacturers is extremely small.

The exception is 'unregulated' mods such as mechanical mods and squonkers, which should not be used by novice vapers. These products do not have safety features such as short circuit protection, overcharge protection or overheating protection.

Child poisoning

Nicotine liquid is potentially toxic and can cause serious harm if ingested, especially in the higher concentrations used for mixing (100mg/mL). Swallowing liquid nicotine is usually followed by intense vomiting and fortunately most cases result in little harm. However there have been some tragic deaths due to accidental poisoning.

Great care should be taken to keep nicotine liquid out of the reach of children and pets. Recommendations on safe use include:

- Always keep nicotine liquid in child-resistant containers
- Store in a safe place, inaccessible to children and pets, preferably in a locked cupboard
- Avoid decanting liquid nicotine into food or drink containers
- Concentrated nicotine (100mg/mL) is best stored in the freezer. There are special lockable storage bags available for that purpose from some vape retailers
- Do not mix nicotine when there are children around. It only takes a brief distraction for a child to drink a fatal dose

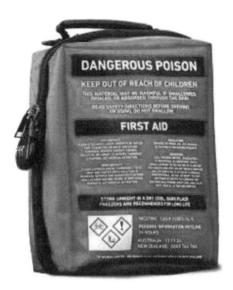

A lockable bag for storing nicotine in the freezer

Safe handling of nicotine

Nicotine liquid can be absorbed through the skin, for example from spills when you refill your device. Large spills or repeated exposure to concentrated nicotine could cause light-headedness, nausea or palpitations. If you spill nicotine liquid on your skin, be sure to wash it off promptly with warm, soapy water.

However, accidental spills over small areas of the fingers or hands are highly unlikely to be a serious health concern[58] and reports of harm from skin contact are extremely rare.[134]

It is good practice to use disposable gloves when handling highly concentrated nicotine solutions. Goggles can help to avoid exposure from splashes to the eyes.

E-liquids

Only buy e-liquids from reputable suppliers. When ordering from overseas vendors you should ask if the products are compliant with the Australian standards.[118]

Black-market producers have no accountability. There is no guarantee that illicit products contain what they claim and there is no assurance of quality or safety.

Do not add any substances that are not intended by the manufacturer, particularly THC (cannabis) oil, which can cause serious lung damage.[87]

Long-term use

Any decision to vape long-term involves weighing up the risks and benefits of vaping and making an informed choice.

Vaping is far safer than smoking, but still involves some risk. Nothing is as safe as breathing fresh air. However, if vaping is helping to stop you going back to smoking, it makes good sense to continue as long as you need to.

Vaping nicotine may also be giving you other positive effects such as improved weight control, temporary stress relief and better concentration. Take all these factors into account in making your decision.

Battery safety

Lithium-ion batteries can malfunction and can cause serious injuries. These events are exceedingly rare as most modern vape devices have a chipset which provides electrical protection and cuts off the power if a problem is detected. The risk of malfunction and harm is even lower from built-in batteries in cigalikes, pod vapes and vape pens.

Nearly all 'exploding e-cigarette' stories you hear about on the news aren't from regulated, properly handled vaping products. They are mostly from loose spare batteries being carried around in a pocket or purse where they come into contact with metal objects like keys or coins and discharge accidentally.

When you fly, vaping devices and spare batteries should always be carried onto the plane in your cabin bag, not stored in your checked luggage. They must not be used, turned on or charged onboard.

Charging your device

When charging your vaping device, make sure that the device, cable, charging adapter and power source are compatible electrically.

Devices with built-in batteries are charged via the USB port (micro-USB or USB C) on the device. Always use the supplied USB cable as the amp rating of the cable matches the specifications of your device. Connect the other end to a low output power source.

It is safe to plug the USB cable into a computer, TV or game console as they provide a low, steady electrical output. Car chargers in the lighter plug are generally safe if the adapter plug operates at 1 amp or less.

If connecting to a wall outlet (the mains power) it is important to use the right USB wall charging adapter (plug). The adapter output should not exceed the maximum charging current your vape can handle.

All adapters sold in Australia are required to have their maximum output written on them in amps. The higher the amp rating, the faster the adapter will charge. Outputs typically range from 0.25-3 amps. All USB devices operate at 5 volts. Good quality low amp (0.5-1 amp) USB wall adapters are generally safe and can be purchased from some vape vendors or other suppliers.

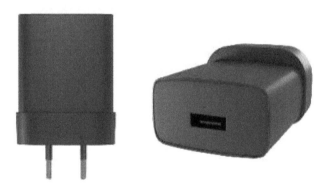

Low amp (0.5-1 amp / 5 volt) wall-to-USB adapters

Check the manual for your vaping device for the recommended maximum charging current, usually 0.5-1 amp (500-1000 milliamps).

Phone and tablet chargers are generally not suitable for charging vapes as almost all are rated ≥2 amps output and deliver too much current. Do not use a wall adapter rated 2 amps if your device's maximum input is 1 amp as this may lead to overheating and battery damage. Fast chargers are especially unsuitable.

Do not keep your device on charge for longer than necessary and never leave it unattended when charging. Charge the device on a non-flammable surface in case of overheating. Check the device from time to time to make sure it is not getting hot.

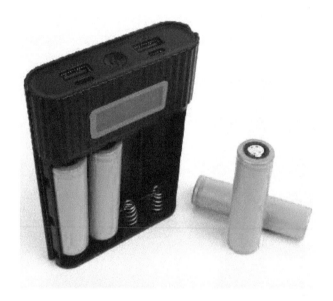

External battery charger with 18650 batteries

Removable battery safety

Removable batteries are very safe to use if properly looked after. Here are some important safety tips to reduce the risk of harm:

- Never keep unprotected, loose batteries in a pocket or purse. Always keep spare batteries in a plastic case and away from metal objects.

- Removable batteries should always be charged in a good quality, dedicated battery charger rather than in the vaping device. An external charger is faster and much safer to use. Using a charger also allows you to have one battery in the vape and another charging at the same time so you always have a charged battery available.

- Always place the battery charger on a non-flammable surface when charging in case of an electrical mishap.

- Only use reputable battery brands from trusted suppliers. Counterfeit copies of brand-name batteries are quite common. It is worth paying a little extra to be sure you are getting the real thing.

- Don't leave your batteries unattended while charging.

- Most chargers have an automatic shut off function to avoid overcharging but it is best to remove the batteries when fully charged.

- Never buy recycled batteries or reclaimed batteries, for example batteries taken from a dismantled laptop.

- Batteries have a protective layer to help prevent short circuits and power leakage. If the cover is damaged, the battery should be discarded or rewrapped with a new wrapping. Your local vape shop should sell new battery wraps and can show you how to do this.

- Do not buy rewrapped batteries.

- Avoid exposing your batteries to extreme temperatures, such as direct sunlight or a car glove box.

- Replace the batteries if they get damaged or wet.

- Batteries for a 2-battery box mod are 'married in pairs' and should always be used together. They should be discharged together at the same time and charged together at the same time.

- Always discard batteries safely into battery recycling containers, not into general rubbish bins. These are available at most vape shops.

- More advanced users should learn more about battery use, understand the 'maximum continuous current' rating of a battery (amp limit) and Ohm's law. A comprehensive resource for geeks is at www.batteryuniverse.com.

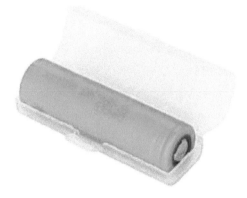

Plastic case for an 18650 battery

Vapor Man

Vapor Man is a vaping activist in his thirties from Melbourne who contacted me in 2020 after the federal Government threatened vapers with a $222,000 fine for importing nicotine.

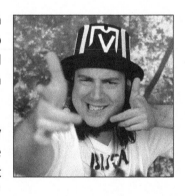

'It's absolutely ridiculous and medievally insane,' he wrote. 'It would be like selling cocaine at every supermarket but requiring a prescription for coffee.'

He began smoking relatively late, at the age of twenty-one at university. 'I knew smoking was bad for me. It certainly wasn't advertisements or ignorance that got me hooked ... possibly hubris. Ever since then, every last smoke in every pack was my last one. I smoked a pack a day for over ten years.'

'At one point I had quit for over a year, but I was constantly irritable and anxious. It was a constant nightmare, with temptation in every corner store, supermarket and social gathering. I started smoking again in one moment of weakness.'

'I tried multiple quitting aids. Fruit flavoured nicotine gum caused horrible indigestion and heartburn and Champix caused suicidal levels of depression.'

Vapor Man switched to vaping six years ago, starting with a box mod and mixing his own e-liquids. Apple pie was the flavour that 'saved me from my own personal hell.' He still uses a box mod with 4mg/mL nicotine.

The benefits have been obvious. 'When I was a smoker I couldn't walk a flight of steps without losing my breath. Now I can vape all day and run thirteen kilometres at night.' There have been huge cost savings. 'I have an espresso machine at home. My one coffee a day actually costs more than my nicotine habit these days.'

'I thought vaping would eventually be promoted as the greatest quitting aid ever invented.' Instead, he was dismayed by the inaccurate and misleading reporting in the media and decided to take action via his YouTube channel. 'That's when I contacted you for help, Doc, I couldn't just sit back and hope it would all work itself out, there's just too much at stake.'

Vapor Man's advice? 'If you're a smoker and you've tried everything else, give it a go. Physically, emotionally, and financially, vaping gave me my life back, and it's not for sale by any stretch.'

Visit Vapor Man's very entertaining YouTube channel at https://tinyurl.com/ajzw4tb9

15

YOU CAN DO IT!

Quitting smoking is one of the hardest challenges you will ever face, but you already know that. You have tried and failed repeatedly with the available treatments and may be wondering if you will ever be able to quit.

Vaping is not a 'silver bullet' and does not work for everyone. But vaping has helped millions of smokers to quit and it could be a lifesaver for you.

Like nicotine patches and gum, vaping replaces the nicotine you crave from smoking. However, unlike other treatments, it replicates the familiar hand-to-mouth action and sensations of smoking. You can continue to enjoy the routine and ritual of being a smoker which can be so hard to give up.

Vaping nicotine is strongly supported by a growing body of scientific research, is endorsed by numerous prestigious international health and medical organisations and is promoted by governments including the United Kingdom, New Zealand and French health authorities. See the Appendix for a list of these.

Vaping is not risk-free and is not for non-smokers or young people. Non-smokers who take up vaping will be increasing their exposure to toxic chemicals, albeit in very low doses.

Vaping is an effective quitting aid

It is no surprise that vaping is the most popular quitting method in Australia and the rest of the world. It is significantly more effective than nicotine replacement therapy and is contributing to an accelerated decline in smoking rates in many countries where it is widely available. Quit rates are even higher with daily use, modern devices and when vaping is combined with counselling and nicotine patches if needed.

While there is continuing debate about youth vaping, there is clear scientific agreement that if you are already smoking, switching to vaping will lead to substantial and immediate health improvements. You will be exposed to dramatically fewer toxic chemicals; your risk of smoking-related diseases will reduce and you will feel and smell better.

These are not idle claims but are backed by abundant scientific evidence and reports from leading health organisations such as the UK Royal College of Physicians and the peak US National Academies of Sciences, Engineering and Medicine.

Just as important for many smokers is the huge financial saving from switching to vaping. Today, the most common reason for wanting to quit is the cost of smoking. Switching to vaping will save you thousands of dollars every year. Imagine what you could do with this extra money!

Misinformation is rampant

Australian opponents of vaping have conducted a successful misinformation campaign to create fear and doubt about vaping. Alarmist and misleading media reports and continuous attacks from government and health bodies have distorted the public perceptions of vaping nicotine.

Just to be clear:

- Vaping is not harmless, but it is at least 95% safer than smoking
- Vaping is significantly more effective as a quitting aid than nicotine patches and gum
- Nicotine creates dependence but has only minor harmful health effects in the doses used in vaping and nicotine has many positive benefits
- The exact long-term risks of vaping nicotine are not known but are certain to be far less than smoking

- Vaping nicotine is completely legal in Australia if you have a prescription from a doctor

The evidence in favour of vaping nicotine is continuing to grow stronger. Each year, over a thousand peer-reviewed articles on vaping are published in medical and scientific journals.[203] We will look back in twenty years and wonder why vaping was not embraced earlier.

Time to make the switch

Quitting smoking is urgent. After the age of thirty-five years, you lose three months of life expectancy permanently for every year you continue to smoke.

However, switching to vaping after years of smoking is a big adjustment and there is a lot to learn. Vape shop staff, online forums, Facebook groups and your doctor are your best sources of expert advice and can help guide you through the journey.

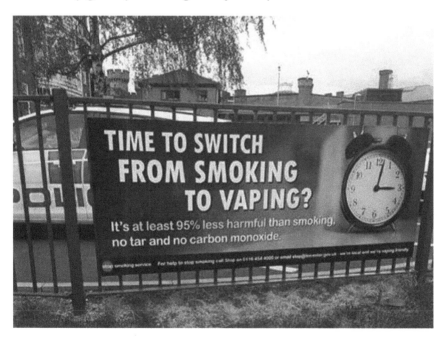

A sign in the UK encouraging smokers to switch to vaping

However even after doing your research, switching is often a matter of trial and error. Don't be afraid to experiment with different vaping devices, e-liquids and nicotine concentrations until you find the right combination.

Sometimes switching to vaping is immediately successful. Sometimes it takes longer. It's safe to keep smoking and vaping until you are ready to quit smoking, gradually reducing and finally quitting cigarettes altogether. Keep trying and check in with the experts when needed.

Don't be afraid to use more nicotine if you are not satisfied. Remember nicotine is not the problem. Almost all the harm from smoking is caused by the toxic chemicals in smoke from burning tobacco.

Finally, after you have quit smoking, it is always best to stop vaping as well if you can. Don't worry if you can't. Continuing to vape is always safer than relapsing to smoking.

Be sure to share your experience far and wide. Tell your family, friends, general practitioner, and local members of parliament. Over time, it will be impossible to ignore the positive benefits of vaping and the hostile anti-vaping policies in Australia will change.

If you are a smoker, switching to vaping could be the best thing you have ever done for your health. You will feel better, live longer and save thousands of dollars every year. What are you waiting for?

Eva

Eva is a retired computer scientist from the Blue Mountains, west of Sydney.

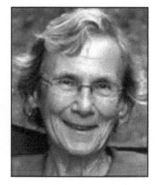

She smoked from the age of fifteen and 'never thought I would be able to quit.' She tried cold turkey a couple of times and used nicotine gums on long-haul flights, all half-heartedly without any conviction.

Ten years ago, Eva retired at the age of sixty-one and realised that she could simply not support her habit on her retirement income.

She researched smoking substitutes on the internet and ordered her first delivery of cigalikes with 18mg/mL nicotine from the US. She was dubious that it would help but was determined to try.

'Despite my doubts, the moment I tried my first e-cig was the moment I stopped smoking. It was nothing short of a miracle!' she said.

'I had no cravings and no withdrawal symptoms of any kind after forty-eight years of smoking. It was as if I had never smoked. Vaping gave me everything I was getting from smoking: nicotine, behaviour, appearance etc., plus the delight of my family (none of whom smoke) and the feeling of achievement.'

'Six months later I tried a single puff of someone else's cigarette and it was horrid beyond words.'

Over ten years, she progressed to refillable pods and DIY liquid with 12mg/mL nicotine content. Her smokers' cough has gone and the gum disease from smoking has improved greatly. She has no intention of give up vaping or reducing her nicotine intake.

Eva estimates she is now saving $12,000 per year. 'I spend about $700 per year on vaping, but cigarettes would be costing me $12,700 per year. If I had kept smoking, I would simply be financially destitute,' she told me.

PART 3

Controversies and solutions

Nicotine vaping is a hotly debated and polarised topic in Australia. Supporters and sceptics both have strong views with intense feelings on each side. Both sides want to reduce the harm from smoking, but there is fundamental disagreement on whether vaping nicotine can play a role.

Traditional public health organisations focus on the risks to young people. Vaping advocates are more concerned about helping established adult smokers quit.

Dr Alex Wodak AM has advocated for drug harm reduction in a number of campaigns over more than thirty years. He explains that 'no matter how impressive the evidence of benefits, or how weak the evidence of serious side effects ... new harm reduction strategies are greeted the same way: with relentless hostility.'[204] Tobacco harm reduction by vaping nicotine is no different.

Part 3 explores the hostile opposition to vaping nicotine in Australia. Why are Australian authorities and most health groups increasingly out of step with other western countries in their resistance to vaping?

It begins with a discussion of youth vaping, the most emotional and highly contested issue followed by a review of the other commonly raised concerns. Most of these concerns are not supported by convincing evidence and many are unfounded.

This has always puzzled me. I naively assumed that once the evidence was clearly outlined, health authorities and policymakers would embrace nicotine vaping.

However, it turns out that much of the opposition is not about the evidence. It is driven more by hidden ideological, moral, political and other agendas. The next section explores how anti-vaping groups defend the indefensible and justify their position without the support of the science.

Other important arguments in favour of vaping are human rights, personal autonomy and social justice and these are also discussed.

This is followed by an outline of how vaping should be regulated in Australia, based on the latest scientific evidence and what works overseas. Regulation needs to allow adult smokers to access high quality vaping products while at the same time minimising access for young people. Getting the balance right between these competing demands is difficult but possible.

The final chapter looks to the future. What can we do to accelerate the necessary changes to vaping policy? A social movement focussing on advocacy, education and political pressure has the best chance of success. Are you willing to take your part?

16

THE RISK TO YOUNG PEOPLE

Take-home messages

- Underage vaping is rare in Australia
- Most adolescent vaping is experimental and infrequent
- Frequently vaping is very rare in teens who have never smoked
- Most adolescents who try vaping are already cigarette smokers
- There is no good evidence that vaping causes young people who would not otherwise have smoked to take up regular smoking
- Vaping is more likely to be a gateway OUT of smoking than INTO smoking
- Nicotine dependence in vaping non-smokers appears to be rare
- Many young people who vape do not use nicotine
- There is no good evidence that nicotine is harmful to the adolescent human brain
- Vaping is far less common and less risky than other substance use by adolescents

Media outlets love the alarmist stories about kids vaping. Nothing gets more clicks from worried parents than the threat of their child becoming instantly addicted to highly toxic chemicals. Apparently, all the kids are doing it. And don't forget it is being pushed by the evil tobacco industry trying to hook a new generation of nicotine addicts. Who wouldn't be terrified of this?

Vaping by young non-smokers is a legitimate concern. There is a risk some will become nicotine-dependent and a very small number may go on to smoking. There are potentially harmful effects from vaping and there is uncertainty about long-term risks. The known risks from vaping are relatively minor but are often greatly exaggerated.

The excessive focus on protecting youth from vaping has led to harsh restrictions which reduce access for adult smokers who are at high risk of near-future disease and death from smoking.[205] It discourages adult smokers who are struggling to quit from trying vaping as a safer alternative.

Disposable nicotine vapes are being sold illegally to young people at tobacconists, retail outlets and on social media. It is hard to understand why authorities claim concern over youth vaping but fail to address illicit sales to underage customers.

Kids should not vape, smoke, binge drink, use illicit drugs or have unsafe sex, but we all know that some will take these risks, no matter what adults tell them. Adolescence is a time of increased risk-taking and sensation-seeking. Young people are attracted to adult products and have accessed cigarettes for generations.

How common is youth vaping?

Media headlines often claim that there is an 'epidemic' of teen vaping in Australia. However, official figures show that underage vaping is rare, and frequent vaping is very rare. Less than two per cent of Australian teenagers vaped once or more in 2019 and more than 90% had never tried vaping.[5]

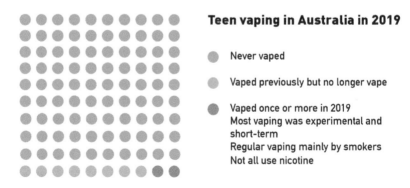

Teen vaping in Australia in 2019

- Never vaped
- Vaped previously but no longer vape
- Vaped once or more in 2019
  Most vaping was experimental and short-term
  Regular vaping mainly by smokers
  Not all use nicotine

Teen (14-17 year old) vaping rates in Australia in 2019[6]

Even these figures exaggerate the issue as most vaping by young people is infrequent and short-term. Of Australian teens who try vaping, one in three do it only once or twice and over 70% do it out of curiosity.[5]

How common is frequent vaping by non-smokers?

Importantly, frequent vaping by non-smokers is very rare. In 2017 (the most recent Australia data) only 0.3% of twelve to seventeen-year-old non-smokers vaped on three or more days in the last month.[206]

Regular vaping by young non-smokers is also rare in other western countries, for example it is < 0.5% in New Zealand,[207] the UK[208] and the US.[209]

Frequent vaping is mostly by teens who already smoke. For them, vaping is likely to be beneficial.

Smoking usually comes first

Most teens who try vaping are already smokers. In 2017, two in three twelve to seventeen year-olds who had vaped in the last month had smoked first, according to the 2017 Australian Secondary Students' Alcohol and Drug Survey.[206]

Surveys in other countries have found that over three in four smoking youth had smoked cigarettes before trying vaping.[153, 210, 211]

In many cases, vaping is used by Australian teens to help them quit smoking (34%), to cut down on smoking (24%), to help prevent relapse (19%) and as a safer alternative to smoking.[5] If young smokers switch to vaping, that can only be a good thing.

Is vaping a 'gateway' into smoking?

The main fear about youth vaping is the so-called 'gateway theory'. This is the concern that young people who would never have smoked will try vaping and, as a result, will become nicotine dependent and progress to regular cigarette smoking. However, the current evidence does not support this.[212]

Teens who try vaping are more likely to try smoking later than those who do not try vaping.[213] However, just because vaping precedes smoking for these teens does not mean that vaping caused the subsequent smoking.

The most likely explanation for the association between vaping and smoking is that young people who experiment with vaping are more prone to taking risks generally. This is known as having a 'common liability' for risk taking (i.e. 'kids who try stuff, try other stuff').[214] We have good evidence that young people who try vaping are also more likely later to binge drink, drink drive and use illicit drugs.[215] This does not mean that vaping causes binge drinking, drink driving or illicit drug use.

Some young people are also more prone to both vaping and smoking because of other personal characteristics or circumstances such as mental health issues, smoking parents, unfavourable home environments, peer pressure, educational under-achievement, or delinquency. It is these influences that lead to smoking not vaping.

There is also growing evidence that some young people are genetically predisposed to both smoking and vaping.[216,217]

According to the New Zealand Ministry of Health,

'Some people worry that vaping might be a 'gateway' to smoking for young people, but there is no clear evidence for this. Smoking among young people is continuing to decline and most young people who vape are smokers or ex-smokers.'[218]

Public Health England's report on youth vaping in 2018 concluded, 'Never-smokers in the UK who try e-cigarettes are more likely to have tried smoking subsequently than those who have not tried e-cigarettes. A causal link has not been established and neither has progression to regular smoking.'[55]

It is quite possible that vaping may lead some non-smokers to experiment with smoking and an even smaller number may go on to become regular smokers. However, the overall effect is likely to be very small.[219, 220]

Nevertheless, the gateway theory lives on in regular media reports. As Kozlowski and Abrams note, 'despite the evidence for a common underlying liability model having replaced the unproven gateway theory, the mere threat of a gateway can create media headlines.'[221]

Vaping is diverting young people from smoking

The overall evidence suggests that vaping is diverting young people away from smoking and reduces the risk of an adolescent becoming a smoker.

Some young people who would have smoked are taking up vaping instead, and are not turning to smoking. This is known as the 'diversion theory' and is consistent with the rapid decline in youth smoking in the United States and United Kingdom since vaping became popular.[222-224]

Youth smoking in the US declined at an unprecedented rate, precisely when youth vaping rates escalated. The blue line in the figure below shows that the fall in youth smoking accelerated after 2013 when vaping (red line) became popular. The dotted line shows the expected smoking rate without vaping based on the historical smoking average.[225] This is consistent with vaping being a gateway out of smoking.

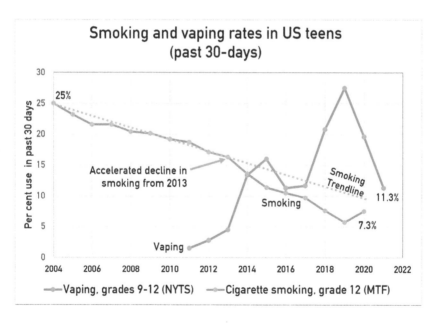

US annual high school (grades 9-12) smoking and vaping rates
Source: US National Youth Tobacco Surveys and Monitoring the Future Surveys

A number of recent studies have demonstrated this diversion effect.

Studies finding that vaping is displacing smoking

1. An analysis of two large national studies in the US over 2014-2020 concluded that, rather than vaping being a gateway to smoking, 'Our results are more consistent with the hypothesis that ECs are displacing young people away from combustible cigarette smoking at the population level.'[226]

2. A study in New Zealand from 2014-19 came to a similar conclusion, that 'the overall decline in smoking over the past six years in New Zealand youth suggests that e-cigarettes might be displacing smoking.'[227]

3. A study found that vaping by non-smokers was most common in those who had previously been identified as having the highest risk of becoming smokers, 'suggesting that e-cigarettes may have replaced smoking'.[228]

4. A study of US high school students found that those who tried vaping first (before smoking) were less likely to be smokers later than those who tried smoking first, suggesting that vaping may have diverted them from becoming smokers.[229]

Further evidence that vaping is a substitute for smoking has come from bans on the sale of vaping products to minors. Teen smoking rates increased significantly after the bans were introduced.[165, 166]

The growing evidence suggests that, even if vaping causes some young people to try smoking, the overall effect is that youth vaping is leading more adolescents away from smoking than towards it.

Are young people becoming 'addicted' to nicotine?

It is rare for young people who have never previously smoked to develop nicotine dependence from vaping although it does occur in some cases. There are several reasons for this:

1. Many young vapers do not use nicotine. Australian data is not available, but national surveys in the US, UK and Norway have found that between 30-70% of young people use flavourings or cannabis only.[230-232] Nicotine use is even less common in young people who vape but do not smoke.

2. Vaping nicotine is less dependence-forming than smoking.[62]

3. Most non-smokers vape infrequently. Infrequent users are less likely to develop nicotine dependence than regular users.

Studies on youth nicotine dependence from vaping

1. In a large national survey in the United States from 2017-19, only 3% of young non-smokers who vaped reported being nicotine dependent (smoking within thirty minutes of waking).[211] The authors of the study concluded, 'Among current e-cigarette users who had never tried tobacco products, responses consistently pointed to minimal dependence.'

2. A recent study of US youth using JUUL, a high nicotine (6%) vaping product, reported that 60% had no symptoms of nicotine dependence.[234] The remaining 40% had very mild dependence— on average 1.6 out of 9 symptoms. Many of these were also current or past smokers and may have already been nicotine dependent anyway.

3. A study of 87,000 US high school students from 2012-2019 found that as vaping became more frequent, smoking rates fell and the overall level of nicotine dependence was unchanged.[233]

4. The UK Royal College of Physicians reported in 2021 that 'e-cigarettes do not seem to be a major source of nicotine addiction for young people in the UK to date.'[142]

Does nicotine harm the adolescent brain?

There is no evidence so far that nicotine harms the human brain in adolescence. Concerns of harm to brain development from nicotine are based on rat and mouse studies.[234] However, laboratory tests often use unrealistic doses in an artificial setting and animals often respond differently to humans. Rodents are more sensitive to nicotine than humans. As one review concluded, animal tests generally 'fall far short of being able to predict human responses.'[113] However, further research is needed to identify any possible long-term effect.[235]

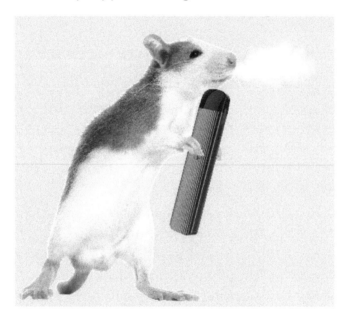

Adolescent mice should not use nicotine

If nicotine is harmful to adolescent brains, we would expect to see some 'epidemiological' evidence for this in the hundreds of millions of adults who smoked when young compared to never-smokers. However, no evidence has been found.

Adolescents are not legally allowed to vape nicotine, but nicotine patches and gum are approved in Australia from the age of twelve and can be purchased from supermarkets and petrol stations.

Is vaping harmful to adolescents?

Adolescents should not vape or smoke. Vaping is not risk-free (nothing is!). It exposes adolescents to low levels of some toxic chemicals and there is some evidence that it may worsen asthma and cause cough and lung irritation in non-smokers.[107] There is a low risk of becoming dependent on nicotine. The risks are less with infrequent vaping which is the main pattern of use.

There are also potential unknown long-term risks from vaping, but significant harms are unlikely, even if use continues for some years. Nearly all lasting harmful effects from smoking can be avoided by quitting before the age of thirty-five years.[236] As vaping is far less risky than smoking, any permanent harm is likely to be delayed even longer and would be much less.

The risk from vaping also needs to be balanced against the diversion of would-be smokers, as discussed above.

Vaping could also have other beneficial effects for adolescents. Vaping could save the lives of their smoking parents and lead to huge financial savings for the family. Adult smokers who switch to vaping and model a healthier behaviour are better role models for their children and reduce their exposure to second-hand smoke.

Is vaping a short-term fad?

Teen fads come and go as young people follow the next cool thing. Kids are programmed to rebel, look for new sensations or do what their peers are doing. Vaping nicotine will be yet another of these, just like Pokémon GO, fidget spinners, car surfing, fad diets and fashions, internet chat rooms, Myspace and even Facebook.

Vaping is likely to be no different. In the US, vaping by year 12 students peaked at 27.5% in 2019 and declined by a huge 60% by 2021 (to 11.3%).[237,238]

Comparison with other youth substance use

Vaping should be viewed in the wider context of teenage risk-taking. During this time of experimentation, there are higher rates of smoking, binge drinking, illicit drug use and unsafe sex to name just a few risky activities, which are a far more serious risk to health.

Alcohol is the most used drug in adolescence and causes the most harm. In 2017, one in three Australian school students aged twelve to seventeen years drank alcohol in the previous week, according to the 2017 Australian Secondary Students' Alcohol and Drug Survey.[206] Around 12% of students admitted to binge drinking in the previous week (five or more drinks on a single occasion). Around 38% of those who drink reported that they intended to get drunk most or every time they drank.

Heavy drinking can lead to violence, road traffic accidents and unintended pregnancies. Over one in every ten deaths (13%) of Australians aged between fourteen and seventeen is alcohol-related and many more are hospitalised.[239]

Cannabis is the most used illicit drug, with 15% of students using it in the last year and about one in three of these using it regularly (on ten or more occasions).[206]

Use of other drugs is less common, but 13% used inhalants, 5% used ecstasy and 3% used hallucinogens in the past year.[206]

In contrast, 1.8% of fourteen to seventeen-year-olds vaped once or more in the last twelve months in the 2019 national survey.[5] The vast majority of use is experimental and frequent use is confined almost exclusively to smokers and ex-smokers.

This is not to condone vaping in young people but is a reminder to keep it in perspective and in proportion to the harm it causes.[240] It makes more sense to focus our concerns more on the most harmful behaviours and less on vaping.

17

OTHER CONTROVERSIES

Take-home messages

- The precise long-term risks of vaping are yet to be established, but are certain to be far less than smoking
- There is no good evidence that vaping is 'renormalising' smoking
- Vaping is not risk-free, but the overall harm from not adopting vaping is far greater than the risk from vaping itself
- Dependence on vaping is much less than from smoking
- Regular vaping by adults who have never smoked is rare
- 'Dual use' is safer than exclusive smoking and is a common transition phase to quitting
- The health risk from long-term vaping is minor compared to the harm from relapsing to smoking
- Vaping competes directly with cigarettes and is an existential threat to cigarette sales

In addition to concerns about youth vaping, opponents of vaping have raised legitimate fears of other possible risks, and these are addressed in this chapter. The anti-vaping case is largely based on theoretical and potential risks which mostly do not survive an objective analysis of the evidence. Not only are the risks often exaggerated but the huge health and financial benefits of switching for adult smokers are mostly ignored.

It is no surprise that most people incorrectly believe that vaping is equally harmful or more harmful than smoking.

'We don't know the long-term risks'

Like all new products, the precise long-term health effects of vaping nicotine will not be known for decades. We do not know everything yet about vaping but we know a lot. Every year, over a thousand peer-reviewed scientific studies on vaping nicotine are published.[203] We also have fifteen years of real-world experience to guide us and there are currently an estimated 68 million people vaping in dozens of countries.[29]

Opponents argue that we should wait another thirty years to be sure about long-term risk. However, this is a double standard not used for any other medicine or treatment. If we applied this standard to medicines, no new treatments would be introduced until we had safety data from thirty years of use.

According to Professor Katherine Baicker, Dean of the Harris School of Public Policy at the University of Chicago, 'Waiting for that level of certainty would paralyse the policy process.'[241] In health policy, she writes 'it is often necessary to act on the basis of the best evidence on hand', even when it is incomplete. 'Doing so requires weighing the costs of acting when you shouldn't against those of not acting when you should.'[241]

Even after allowing for potential unknown risks, the UK Royal College of Physicians has estimated that the long-term risk of vaping is unlikely to be more than 5% of the risk of smoking.[12]

The unreasonable requirement for long-term proof was not applied to Covid-19 vaccines. The Australian government approved vaccines (rightly) after only months of research but requires decades more research on vaping. However, less than 1,000 Australians died from Covid-19 in 2020 and over 21,000 die prematurely every year from smoking.

As with any new product, it is possible that some harms may emerge over time and monitoring of vaping should continue in order to detect any new side-effects.

'Vaping is not completely safe'

Nothing is completely safe, but some vaping opponents demand absolute safety from vaping before they will accept it.[242] For example, the president of the Australian Medical Association told the Parliamentary Inquiry into the Use of Electronic Cigarettes and Personal Vaporisers in 2017 that he would not consider vaping unless it was shown to be 100% harmless.[243] This is an unrealistic standard which is not applied to anything else.

The real question is not whether vaping is 100% safe but whether it is safer than smoking ('relative risk'). Vaping is a substitute for smokers who would otherwise be smoking. There is universal agreement that vaping is far less risky than smoking.

Some non-smokers who may never have smoked may take up vaping, but research suggests this number is very small indeed and the number going on to regular smoking is even smaller. It is unreasonable to withhold a life-saving tool for millions of adult smokers because some non-smokers may misuse it and be exposed to a minor risk.

'But it took decades to find out that smoking was harmful'

If cigarettes were invented today, we would know very quickly that they are very harmful.

We know much more today about chemistry, toxicology, physiology and the causes of disease than when cigarettes were introduced over a century ago. We have a much greater understanding of the harmful effects of most chemicals and can assess them against occupational and environmental health and safety standards. The scientific method, analytical techniques, and equipment available now are far superior to those used in the past.

Our understanding of vaping and its health effects is rising exponentially.[203]

'Vaping will renormalise smoking'

Vaping critics fear that widespread vaping could 'renormalise' smoking. They worry vaping may make smoking appear more socially acceptable and that this could undermine decades of successful tobacco control efforts. However, there is no evidence that this is happening in other countries and some evidence that vaping may be de-normalising smoking.

According to Public Health England,

'There is no evidence that ENDS (vaping products) are undermining the long-term decline in cigarette smoking among adults and youth and may in fact be contributing to it.'[84]

The UK Royal College of Physicians concluded, 'There is no evidence that … e-cigarette use has resulted in renormalisation of smoking.[12] Instead, 'e-cigarettes have … helped to de-normalise tobacco use.'[142]

The New Zealand Ministry of Health came to the same conclusion, 'There is no international evidence that vaping products are undermining the long-term decline in cigarette smoking among adults and youth, and may in fact be contributing to it'.[244]

The main sign of renormalisation would be stagnating or rising smoking rates.[245] In fact, the opposite is occurring. The decline in smoking rates has accelerated in the UK and US since vaping became widely available. In Australia, where vaping is discouraged, smoking rates are declining much more slowly.

'People will get addicted to nicotine'

Almost all vapers are already dependent on nicotine from past smoking and have transferred their nicotine dependence to a much safer product. Smokers who switch to vaping become less dependent and find it easier to quit vaping when they are ready to try.[62] Very few non-smokers become regular vapers. In Australia, only 0.2% of non-smokers were vaping monthly or more in 2019.[5]

Smoking is particularly addictive because it delivers high levels of nicotine very rapidly to the brain. Vaping releases nicotine more slowly and generally to lower levels. Smoke also contains other chemicals that make nicotine more addictive, for example, monoamine oxidase inhibitors.[129] These chemicals are not present in vapour.

Non-smokers who try vaping are also less likely to use nicotine. In the UK, 41% of adult smokers who vaped reported using nicotine compared to 7% of those who had never smoked.[246]

Many vapers do not regard dependence on nicotine from vaping as a problem. Nicotine has many positive and pleasurable effects and is a relatively benign substance in the doses used.

'We should follow the precautionary principle'

Some vaping sceptics argue that there are things we don't know about vaping, so it is better to wait until we have more information. 'Better to be safe than sorry.' This is known as the 'precautionary principle'.[247]

However, the precautionary principle is misused when applied to vaping.[248] Applying the precautionary principle requires weighing the risks of allowing vaping against the risks of not allowing it. Easier access to vaping has small and theoretical risks but the harm from overcautious regulation is much greater, as it denies many smokers the opportunity to quit or switch to a potentially life-saving product.

In the absence of conclusive long-term evidence, one way to estimate the overall impact of vaping is to use 'simulation modelling'. This involves estimating the potential risks of vaping and the potential benefits to predict the overall impact on community health. Numerous modelling studies (with one exception) have concluded that the benefits of vaping are considerably greater than the costs.[249, 250]

After taking the risks of vaping into account, one study projected that replacing most smoking with vaping in the US over a ten-year period would result in averting between 1.6-6.6 million premature deaths and between 20.8 – 86.7 million fewer life-years lost.[251]

'Non-smoking adults will take up vaping'

Vaping is largely confined to smokers and ex-smokers and regular use by adults who have never smoked is rare.

In Australia in 2019, less than one in a hundred adult non-smokers vaped once or more in the previous twelve months.[5] In most cases, vaping by non-smokers is experimental and short-term, often does not involve nicotine and rarely becomes regular use.

According to the New Zealand Ministry of Health in 2020,

> 'Despite some experimentation with vaping products among never smokers, vaping products are attracting very few people who have never smoked into regular vaping, including young people.' [244]

Public Health England reported in 2021 that only 0.2-0.6% of adults in the UK who had never smoked were currently vaping. Never-smokers also vaped less frequently than current or former smokers and most (57%) tried vaping only once or twice.[46]

Other international surveys have found that vaping by adult non-smokers is generally less than half of one percent of the adult population, for example in the United States 0.3%[160]; Germany 0.3%[252]; Iceland 0.4%[253]; and Greece 0.2%.[254] In New Zealand there was no regular use reported by adult non-smokers[255] and current daily vaping by never smokers in the European Union was 0.08%.[256]

'Vapers will keep smoking as well (dual use)'

Critics are concerned that some smokers will smoke and vape at the same time ('dual use') instead of quitting smoking. In Australia, just over half of all vapers were also smoking in 2019.[5] However, dual use is a normal, temporary transition phase for most smokers and many go on to quitting.[257,258]

Some smokers quit smoking soon after they start vaping. Others take longer and smoke and vape for a period while trying to transition to exclusive vaping. Some return to exclusive smoking. This is to be expected as dual users are heavier smokers and are more addicted.[259,260] Most studies show that dual users are also more likely to quit smoking than exclusive smokers, especially if they vape daily.[261]

Dual use rates decrease over time as smokers adapt to vaping. In Great Britain, the rate of dual use fell from 65% of vapers in 2014 to 30% in 2021[262] and in the US from 57% in 2015 to 41% in 2018.[263] It is very likely that more dual users would switch completely to vaping if public messaging was clear about its far lower risk.

Dual use is less harmful than exclusive smoking because most dual users significantly cut back their smoking.[264] Most studies show dual users have lower levels of toxins in the body compared to smokers[265] and many studies show improvements in health, such as reduced blood pressure[92] and improved asthma control.[110]

The only potential harm from dual use is if it reduces interest in quitting. However, this does not appear to be the case. Smokers who vape are more interested in quitting than those who do not and are more likely to make quit attempts.[266]

'Many continue to vape long-term'

It is recommended that users stop vaping after they have successfully quit smoking. However, for many former smokers, relapse is a constant threat. Research suggests that continuing to vape can help to prevent relapse.[10] Vaping can act as a replacement for smoking behaviour to help cope with urges to smoke.

The health risk from continuing to vape is minor compared to the harm from relapsing to smoking.

'Australia has been very successful in reducing smoking'

Tobacco control strategies such as high taxation and smoking bans have reduced smoking in Australia over the last few decades. However, one in seven adults, or nearly 3 million Australians still smoke[5] and smoking remains Australia's largest preventable killer.[1] Smoking rates remain alarmingly high among disadvantaged groups, such as people on low incomes, Indigenous people and people with mental illness.[5]

Since 2013, the decline in smoking in Australia has slowed significantly[5, 25] and has been one third of the decline over the same period in the UK where vaping is widely available (8% v 25% decline).[164]

Australia's adult daily smoking rate was 13.8% in 2017-18,[268] far behind the goal of 10% set for 2018 in the National Tobacco Strategy 2012-2018.[32]

As outlined in the National Tobacco Strategy, tobacco harm reduction is one of the three pillars of tobacco control, along with strategies for reducing supply and demand.[32] However, it still has not been supported in health policy.

This is not good enough and we need to do better.

'We already have approved aids for quitting smoking'

Conventional aids such as nicotine replacement therapy, varenicline (Champix) and bupropion (Zyban) work for some people. However, the success rates are extremely low. Only 6-15% of smokers in clinical trials have quit after six to twelve months with these treatments[64] and the numbers are even lower in real world use without professional support.[267]

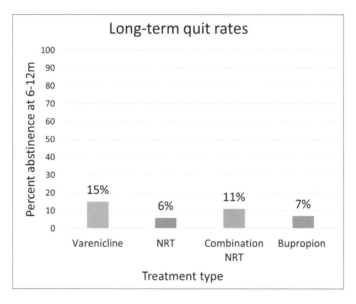

Quit rates from smoking cessation treatments at 6-12 months

Smokers need a range of quitting options to choose from as different methods suit different people.

The traditional quitting medicines are also underused.[5] This may be because of concerns about safety, low success rates, restricted access to medical care, resistance to the 'medicalisation' of smoking or thinking that you should be able to do it on your own.

In contrast, vaping has considerable appeal to smokers. Vaping is the most popular quitting aid in Australia and the rest of the world because it replicates the smoking experience with only a fraction of the toxins. It is also a pleasurable activity, allowing the smoker to continue to enjoy nicotine.

'Vaping is a tobacco company plot to keep people smoking'

Some anti-vaping advocates like to position vaping nicotine as a tobacco industry conspiracy. They claim that the tobacco industry's aim is 'to hook kids to smoking,' 'to keep more adults smoking' or 'undermine tobacco control.'

This is a compelling argument because of the tobacco industry's appalling and dishonest reputation. However, the real story is quite different.

Modern vaping devices were invented as a quitting aid in 2003 by a Chinese chemist, Hon Lik. Mr Hon was a two-pack-a-day smoker who was unable to quit with other methods. Like so many people after him, he quit smoking with vaping.

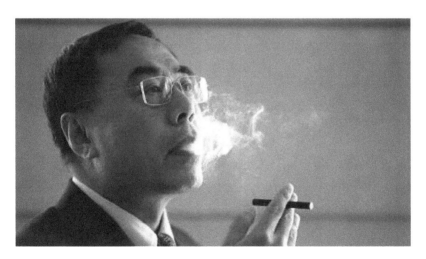

Hon Lik, the inventor of the modern e-cigarette

Mr Hon's invention is a huge disruptive threat to the tobacco industry. Vaping products are in direct competition with cigarettes. Vaping is to cigarettes what digital cameras were to Kodak and electric cars are to the combustible engine – an existential threat to survival.

The tobacco industry first invested in vaping in 2012 and it has been trying to catch up ever since. The tobacco industry currently controls no more than 20% of the global vapour market.[29] At present, the tobacco industry does not have any vaping interests in Australia.

As vaping has become more widespread, there has been an unprecedented decline in the value of international tobacco stocks. Share prices fell by more than half from 2017-2020. Proposals to restrict vaping have been repeatedly followed by rises in tobacco stocks and increased cigarette sales.[268]

In the area of tobacco harm reduction, tobacco companies are mostly focussed on heated tobacco products, an alternative reduced-risk smokeless product, rather than vaping products.

If the tobacco industry transitions from making cigarettes to safer nicotine alternatives, that can only be a good thing for society and should be encouraged. Philip Morris's smoke-free nicotine products accounted for 29% of its global net revenue in the second quarter of 2021, compared with 0.2% in 2015, and the proportion is increasing every year.[269]

Many people demand that tobacco companies stop making deadly cigarettes if they are genuine about reducing the harms from smoking. However, all public companies have a legal duty to maximise company profits and a responsibility to shareholders. A CEO who pushed this line would simply be replaced with another who would maintain the business.

It is unscientific to oppose a safer product just because it is associated with tobacco companies. Although we can't trust the tobacco industry based on their past behaviour, our overriding priority should be to reduce the death and disease caused by tobacco use as quickly as possible. Safer alternatives to smoking will save lives, regardless of who makes them.

18

MISPERCEPTIONS ABOUT SAFETY

Take-home messages

- Beliefs about the harms of vaping are exaggerated
- We do not make rational decisions about risk
- Decisions are automatic, subconscious
- Emotions influence our decision-making more than logical thinking
- Media reporting distorts the real risk
- We should compare the risk of vaping to smoking, assess the absolute risk and probability, assess if the risk is real and consider the benefits of vaping

We like to think we make rational decisions when estimating the risks of everyday activities. However, we often get it wrong.

For example, panic about the extremely rare risk of blood clots from the AstraZeneca vaccine for Covid-19 led to delays in the vaccination rollout in Australia and some other countries with potentially deadly outcomes. Many people also have an exaggerated fear of shark attacks. Although a terrifying prospect, the actual risk of dying from such an event in Australia is about one in 8 million each year – a tiny risk by any standard.

Most people also overestimate the harms of vaping. In the UK in 2021, only 12% of those surveyed correctly believed that it was much less harmful than smoking.[270]

Furthermore, the misperceptions of vaping harm are increasing. In the US, the proportion of US adults who thought e-cigarettes were equally or more harmful than cigarettes increased from 53.7% to 72.7% from 2013 to 2016.[271]

In Australia, misperceptions about the safety of vaping may be partly due to a lack of support from government agencies, health bodies and charities and constant negative messaging designed to discourage its use.[272]

Why do we get it wrong?

Why do intelligent people come to irrational conclusions about the harm of vaping?

According to Nobel laureate Daniel Kahneman, we are far less rational than we think we are.[273] In his book, *Thinking, Fast and Slow* he explains how our minds are riddled with biases leading to poor decision-making. Much of our thinking is intuitive, automatic and subconscious ('fast thinking').

When making quick decisions, we often make shortcuts and jump to unsound conclusions which fit with our prior beliefs. We think we've considered all the relevant factors and are making the optimal choice. However, the brain fails to realise that evidence is missing and does not weigh evidence appropriately. People often give too much weight to small risks and tend to be overly confident about their beliefs. These first impressions carry a lot of weight and are hard to shift.

The process of fast thinking is an evolutionary survival skill. Fast thinking helps us to react quickly and automatically and avoid being eaten by a lion!

'Another part of our brain' analyses information more logically and slowly ('slow thinking'). This type of thinking requires more effort and conscious reasoning but often doesn't get used. Laziness is built into our nature, and we follow the path of least effort. Kahneman found in his studies that people often ignore the statistical facts and hard evidence in their decision making.

The role of the media

How the media covers vaping influences our perceptions of the risk from vaping.

The media gives prominence to negative reports on vaping which create an exaggerated sense of risk.[274] For example, a study of US news articles on vaping from 2015 to 2018 found that 70% of the articles mentioned vaping's risk for youths, while only 37% noted potential benefits for adult smokers.[31]

Alarmist reports of a youth vaping 'epidemic', malfunctioning vaping devices and rare cases of child poisoning are more click-worthy than the inspiring stories of people whose lives have been transformed by vaping or positive findings from research.

News media tend to pay special attention to the emotional aspects of a story and select issues that generate strong primal emotions, such as fear, worry and dread.[274,275] Our automatic, emotional response to a story has more impact on our risk perceptions than our logical thinking, even when the probability of an event is low. Our response overrides our rational judgement and magnifies our fears.

Our brains have learned to give priority to danger and this has served us well as a survival strategy. We instinctively pay more attention to reports of risk and danger, forming critical first impressions well before we have all the facts. First assessments are hard wired and are fiercely held despite later evidence to the contrary. This creates a 'perception gap' in which our irrational fears do not match the facts.[275]

How the media presents or 'frames' a risk is very influential.[274] Framing involves selecting and highlighting certain aspects of a story to promote a particular interpretation. Media reports often emphasise the dramatic aspects of a story which amplify the public's perception of risk.

Kahneman also found that people judge the importance of issues by how easy they are to retrieve from the memory.[273] Frequent coverage of emotional and dramatic stories is easily recalled and strongly influences our perception of risk. It is easier to recall reports of exploding vapes than stories of the millions of peoples who have quietly saved their lives by vaping.

How to assess the risk of vaping

To assess the risk from vaping, we need to use our conscious mind to examine the evidence. Ask these questions when reading a media report on a risk from vaping:[276]

1. How does the risk compare to smoking (relative risk)?

The risk from vaping should always be compared to the behaviour it replaces, tobacco smoking ('relative risk'). Almost all vaping is by smokers or former smokers who would otherwise be smoking.

2. How large is the risk (the absolute risk)?

Vaping is not harmless, but the level of risk is very low.

3. How likely is the risk to occur (probability)?

Isolated reports of rare events create the impression that an issue is more common than it really is. Serious harm from vaping nicotine is extremely rare.

4. Is the risk real?

Be cautious of animal and cell studies, and reports of trace amounts of chemicals in vaping products. If a biological effect or toxic chemical is identified, is it likely to cause material harm or disease in humans?

5. Does the risk justify the benefits of the activity?

The small and potential risks of vaping should be weighed against the substantial health benefits and the pleasure it gives.

6. Was smoking the cause?

If a health concern is identified, could it be due to past smoking. Almost all vapers are former smokers.

19

HOW ARE INDIVIDUAL ATTITUDES TO VAPING FORMED?

Take-home messages

- Initial attitudes to vaping are often based on instinctive and morally driven views
- Attitudes are justified later by more socially acceptable reasons
- Once a strong position is formed, it is maintained by confirmation bias
- False beliefs become even more entrenched when confronted with the facts (the backfire effect)

Why is the debate on vaping so polarised? How can rational individuals, on both sides reach opposing and unshakeable conclusions from the same evidence? A key factor in shaping our views is what is known as 'moral psychology'.

Moral psychology

In his book *The Righteous Mind: Why Good People are Divided by Politics and Religion,* psychologist Jonathan Haidt explains that initial attitudes are formed quickly and are instinctively and morally driven, rather than based on an evaluation of the relevant evidence.[277]

Initial and emotional reactions are 'so fast and compelling that they act like blinders on a horse'. Later, people or organisations selectively look for evidence to justify their positions. As Haidt explains, 'Intuitions come first, strategic reasoning second.'[277]

For example, a person may hold a subconscious belief that 'using an addictive substance is sinful' or 'new technologies can't be trusted' or may see vaping as a threat to their self-interest. This could generate an immediate negative attitude to vaping nicotine.

Justifying beliefs

Haidt says people, 'have strong gut feelings about what is right or wrong ... and construct post hoc justifications for those feelings.' The 'gut reaction' against vaping could later be justified publicly by a more socially acceptable but false argument, such as 'vaping is leading young people to take up smoking.' This use of moral psychology is a well-accepted phenomenon in harm reduction debates.[278]

Rationalisations based on 'protecting our children' or 'fighting the evil tobacco industry' are especially powerful because of their emotional impact and the moral panic they create.

Why we rarely change attitudes

Once we form a strong opinion on a complex moral issue like vaping, we desperately cling to it. We look for evidence that supports it, which we accept at face value, while quickly dismissing evidence that contradicts it. This is known as confirmation bias.[279]

Or, as Haidt explains, in reading research with inconvenient findings, 'It's always possible to question the methods, find an alternative explanation of the data, or, if all else fails question the honesty or ideology of the researchers.'

Once a strong position is established, it is almost impossible to change it by presenting the facts. Haidt says, 'this is why moral and political arguments are so frustrating. You can't change people's minds by utterly refuting their argument.'

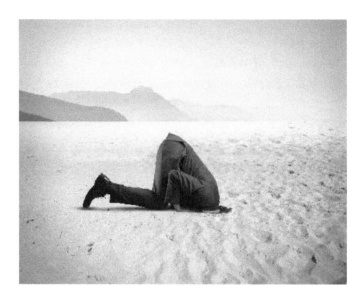

We ignore the evidence that contradicts our predetermined views

Indeed, when confronted with new evidence, false beliefs often become more deeply entrenched (the 'backfire effect').[280] Reasonable attempts at discussion or logical persuasion are generally doomed to failure.[281]

Even scientists interpret evidence in a biased manner to confirm their initial beliefs. According to two leading addiction journal editors, 'we are seeing conclusions being drawn from e-cigarette research that appear to be based in many cases on pre-suppositions rather than a dispassionate analysis of the evidence and its context.'[282]

Following the crowd

Once a false view appears to be widely established in society, such as 'vaping is very harmful', individuals often feel the need to conform to avoid social isolation. This is known as 'conformity bias'.

In his 2021 book, *The Constitution of Knowledge: A Defense of Truth*, journalist Jonathan Rauch explains how we feel pressure to conform to the prevailing view.[420] 'We harmonize our beliefs and even our perceptions with those of the people around us, often without being aware of doing so.'

'Even in the face of countervailing evidence', we are less likely to speak up for fear of criticism, creating a 'spiral of silence'. Our silence increasingly creates the impression that the prevailing opinion is correct.

This human weakness to make and maintain irrational attitudes applies to both sides of the vaping debate but is far more pronounced in those who oppose vaping, in my opinion.

20

TEN UNDERLYING REASONS
WHY VAPING IS OPPOSED

Take-home messages

Disapproval of vaping is largely based on unstated biases, fears and self-interest, such as

- A zero tolerance to smoking and nicotine
- Moral outrage at the immoral use of an 'addictive' drug
- Distrust of tobacco companies
- Vested interests of organisations and individuals
- Minimising political risk and maximising tobacco taxes
- Financial conflicts of interest
- Fear of innovation and new technology
- Belief that nicotine liquid should be a medicine

For decades, tobacco control and public health organisations have sought to stigmatise tobacco, nicotine, smoking and smokers. The invention of vaping, a far safer nicotine alternative which looks like smoking, is a threat to their strongly-held views and the traditional approach.

Attitudes to vaping nicotine are shaped less by the scientific evidence and more by this long-standing prohibitionist approach. Other factors such as moral judgements, values and priorities, politics, vested interests and financial factors also play a role.[272] These considerations help to explain why different organisations have diametrically opposed views, despite using the same evidence.

Australian federal and state governments, Heart Foundation Australia, Cancer Council Australia and the Australian Medical Association oppose vaping nicotine. Their position is in stark contrast to the UK government, the British Heart Foundation, Cancer Research UK and the British Medical Association that support vaping nicotine as an opportunity to save lives.

1 'Abstinence-only' ideology

Australia has been successful in reducing smoking rates by promoting complete abstinence from tobacco and nicotine. **Tobacco harm reduction has not been part of the traditional approach and is seen by some as a threat to it**.

This contrasts with the UK's long-standing support for tobacco harm reduction. The UK Royal College of Physicians published its first report supporting harm reduction for nicotine products in 2007.[283] This was followed by support from the National Institute for Health and Care Excellence in 2013[284] and subsequent reports from the Royal College of Physicians in 2014,[285] 2016[12] and 2021.[142] The 2021 report stated,

> 'On the basis of available evidence, the RCP believes that e-cigarettes could lead to significant falls in the prevalence of smoking in the UK, prevent many deaths and episodes of serious illness, and help to reduce the social inequalities in health that tobacco smoking currently exacerbates.'

Australia's zero tolerance of nicotine is not consistent with our approach to other forms of harm reduction. We accept the use of methadone as a substitute for people who use heroin but not clean forms of nicotine to reduce the harm from smoking, Australia's biggest preventable killer.

It is also not consistent with Australia's National Tobacco Strategy[32] and National Drug Strategy,[286] both of which include a legitimate and integral role for harm reduction strategies.

The goal of tobacco control should be to end the death and suffering from smoking, not to eliminate nicotine from society. Nicotine is part of the problem, but it can also be part of the solution as a harm reduction tool. The 'war on nicotine', just like the war on drugs and other forms of prohibition, is doomed to failure.[287]

2 Moral outrage

Opposition to harm reduction policy has a 'strong underlying tone of moralism' according to distinguished Professor of Public Health, Ken Warner from the University of Michigan.[288]

Some opponents of vaping believe that any use of an 'addictive' substance is wrong. Anything that looks like a cigarette or works like one and delivers nicotine is seen as sinful or immoral and must be eliminated, and this takes priority even when there are substantial health benefits.[278]

Warner notes 'a distinctly puritanical streak within the public health community' that will only accept 'Just say no' when it comes to nicotine.[278] It is especially unacceptable if people get pleasure from vaping nicotine, choose to do it recreationally or if the tobacco industry is involved in some way. The game plan of Big Public Health has been to punish, coerce and stigmatise smokers (and now vapers) until they change their wicked ways.

Moral and emotional arguments are common on issues such as illicit drugs, alcohol, the sex industry and sex outside marriage. For example, a preacher opposed to sex before marriage would be horrified at the prospect of distributing condoms to young people, even though this would prevent pregnancy and sexually transmitted disease. In the same way, the moral objection to vaping nicotine will result in more deaths from smoking.

Moral judgements have a strong influence over public policy on harm reduction. This helps to explain why compelling evidence alone is not be enough to bring about sensible regulations on vaping.[289]

3 Competing values and priorities

Our values, priorities and goals influence how we interpret the evidence. For example, if you believe that even the smallest risk to young people from vaping is not justified at any cost, you will oppose it even if there are substantial and immediate benefits for established adult smokers.

The Thoracic Society of Australia and New Zealand is a vocal opponent of vaping and understandably opposes anything which may harm the lungs.[290] Vaping is not as pure as mountain air and long-term use may cause some harm to the lungs. However, their opposition to vaping nicotine is counterproductive. The harm from smoking is much greater and vaping has the potential to dramatically reduce lung disease in smokers who switch.

Policy decisions involve trade-offs and compromises. Policy on vaping should be based on its overall impact on public health, not on areas of narrow interest. For example, the small potential risk of vaping to young people is dwarfed by the substantial and immediate benefits of quitting by adult smokers. Furthermore, the risk to young people can be minimised with sensible regulation and enforcement.

4 Distrust of the tobacco industry

Tobacco control warriors have long fought a noble crusade to destroy the tobacco companies, whose deadly products kill up to two in three long-term smokers. This industry has repeatedly misled the public, blocked reforms with legal action and put profits before public health. The campaign against Big Tobacco has been driven by science, passion, and the high moral ground.

Since tobacco companies entered the vaping market, the focus of tobacco control shifted to attack vaping to punish the tobacco industry. There is a view that 'If the tobacco companies are involved in vaping, it must be a bad thing and must be opposed'. As Clive Bates explains,

'The war on smoking morphed into a war on nicotine. The machine built for fighting smoking swivelled its gun turrets and

started blasting away at the new products and their supporters...
The leaders grew up as veterans of the 'tobacco wars' and continued their fight on the new fronts.'[291]

However, this is counterproductive as nicotine vaporisers are life-
saving products which compete directly with cigarettes. Furthermore,
the tobacco companies only control a small share of the vaping market.[292] The war against the tobacco industry appears to have taken pre-
cedence over the primary goal of public health, which is to reduce the
death and disease from smoking.

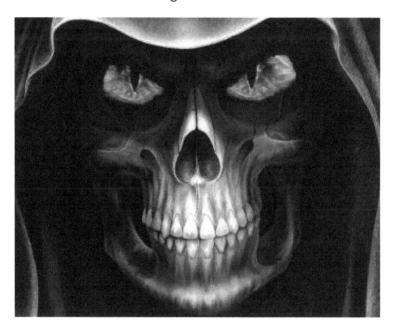

Big Tobacco plays only a small role in vaping

**The tragic irony is that those who oppose vaping are supporting
the very thing they are trying to eradicate – combustible cigarette
sales.** Vaping is a disruptive threat to the very existence of the tobacco
industry, just like renewable energy is to fossil fuels. Attacks on vaping to
punish the cigarette companies perversely lead to more people smoking
and bigger tobacco company profits.[292]

5 Protection of self-interest

Some public health organisations and individuals are threatened by solutions that may reduce their relevance and try to defend the status quo.

Tobacco control organisations have constructed a machine for fighting the tobacco industry and smoking and now they are saying their machine is still needed to fight the new evil, vaping nicotine. Opposing vaping provides a justification for their continuing role.

They have prior positions to defend, organisations to run, funders' interests to respect, and rely on government, pharmaceutical and philanthropic funding to support their ongoing research, conferences, wages and campaigns.

However, instead of improving public health, this strategy has the opposite effect and will undoubtedly undermine their reputations and public confidence in them.[293]

Some tobacco control professionals see vaping nicotine as a threat to their legacy and prestige. Vaping was developed outside the tobacco control movement and pharmaceutical industry and triggers the NIH Syndrome ('not invented here').[294] It is opposed because it was not their idea, and especially because it has the temerity to be so effective. Vaping threatens the abstinence-only narrative they have spent their professional lives promoting.

According to behavioural scientist, Rory Sutherland, in his book, *Alchemy: The Surprising Power of Ideas that Don't Make Sense*, the last thing they want to hear is that 'the problem to which you have dedicated your life and from which your social status derives is no longer a problem anymore.'[295]

Mark Tyndall, Professor in the School of Population and Public Health at the University of British Columbia in Canada goes one step further. He says,

> 'Instead of viewing vaping as a disruptive technology that could actually replace cigarettes, 'tobacco control' advocates see

vaping as a technology that could actually replace them and their abstinence-based programs that are largely ineffective.'[296]

Vaping is a paradigm shift and does not sit well with the traditional strategy of the tobacco control movement.

6 Political risk

Governments are driven by minimising political risk. It is politically safer to take no action on vaping.

Joshua Newman, Professor of Social Sciences at Monash University, Melbourne, wrote about e-cigarette regulation in Australia,

> 'Australian governments have not been following an evidence-based approach and, further ... these governments are instead content to minimise political risk by either taking no action or by adapting existing legislation.'[297]

Since vaping products are used by a relatively small number of voters and public perceptions about vaping are negative, there are few political rewards for proactive regulation. More kudos can be gained by appearing to be 'tough on the tobacco companies' or 'protecting our children'.

Public health policy should always be based on the best available scientific evidence. However, in reality this only seems to occur when the evidence aligns with political objectives.

According to Professor Steve Allsop, former Director at the National Drug Research Institute at Curtin University,

> 'research is about evidence, fidelity and logical argument while politics is about the next election, perceptions, bargains and timing.'[298]

7 Groupthink

Groupthink (or 'tribalism') is 'a phenomenon that occurs when a group of well-intentioned people makes irrational or non-optimal decisions spurred by the urge to conform or the belief that dissent is impossible.'[299]

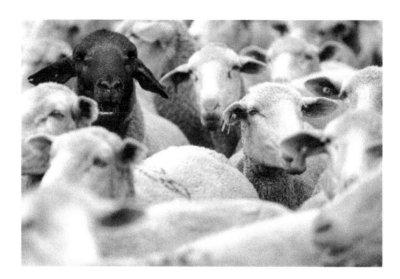

It is safer to follow the flock

Groupthink operates within public health organisations and is a powerful and disruptive force. 'Smart people are vulnerable to putting the tribe before truth,' explains Yale Psychology Professor Dan Kahan.[300] Even smart people with good scientific literacy interpret the evidence selectively to reach a view that is consistent with the views and identity of their tribe. At the same time, they dismiss evidence that undermines the group beliefs.

Compliance is understandable. Taking a contradictory view on vaping risks career and funding opportunities, and disapproval from peers. It is safer to 'follow the flock'.

At a national level, the Australian health organisations are locked in an echo chamber of groupthink on vaping. Organisations typically justify their position based on the support of other groups with similar views.

8 Fear of innovation and new technology

New technologies generate fear and scepticism and are often resisted even when there are substantial benefits.

In the book, *Innovation and Its Enemies: Why People Resist New Technologies*, the late Professor Calestous Juma from Harvard University explains how innovations that are widely accepted today, such as coffee, margarine and refrigeration were ferociously opposed when first introduced. He writes,

> 'Claims about the promise of new technology are at times greeted with scepticism, vilification, or outright opposition – often dominated by slander, innuendo, scare tactics, conspiracy theories, and misinformation. The assumption that new technologies carry unknown risks guides much of the debate. This is often amplified to levels that overshadow the dangers of known risks.'[301]

9 Financial conflicts of interest

Vaping is a serious financial threat to organisations that benefit from tobacco taxes.

Tobacco taxes generated AUD$17.4 billion in Australia in 2019-20, the fourth highest tax after company tax, income tax and GST.[302] As tobacco researcher Dr Carl Phillips notes, 'Governments derive enormous revenue from taxing cigarettes and generally lose that when smokers switch to vaping.'[303]

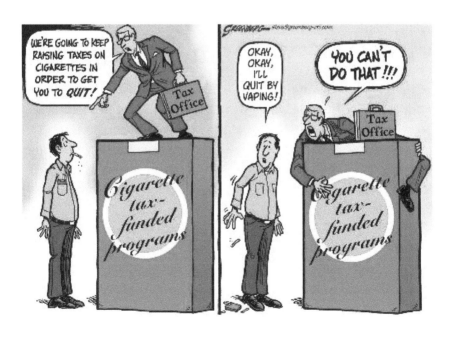

It is often said that the government is addicted to tobacco tax revenue more than people are addicted to smoking.

The Australian government frames tobacco tax increases as a public health strategy. However, most smokers believe it is a cynical tax grab by a greedy government, exploiting and punishing smokers for their addiction.[304] Tobacco taxes are having a diminishing effect on smoking rates at the current eye-watering levels but they certainly help to balance the budget. The vast majority of this money goes into general revenue and only a tiny portion is used to help smokers quit, the stated aim of the policy.

Without combustible products, there is no need for tobacco control organisations. Their existing infrastructure was built on the harms of smoking and it has to find new harms to maintain its relevance and funding.

Phillips says 'The very people who lead anti-smoking efforts have a serious financial conflict of interest about succeeding' and vaping is clearly a threat.[303]

Vaping nicotine is also opposed by Big Pharma in Australia. Vaping improves health and reduces the need for medicines generally and stop-smoking medication in particular.

In the US in 1998, forty-six states and some territories came to an agreement with the tobacco industry called the Master Settlement Agreement (MSA).[305] The industry agreed to pay the states each year a sum based on their smoking rate to compensate for the costs of treating sick and dying smokers. Some states arranged to borrow against this future income stream but got into difficulties when the decline in smoking rates fell faster than anticipated after vaping became popular. The states with the greatest resulting financial debt are also the very states most hostile to vaping.

Funding of organisations by philanthropists can also influence policy. Billionaire Michael Bloomberg is strongly opposed to vaping and funds a range of organisations which support his agenda, such as the World Health Organisation and Tobacco Free Kids in the US. Many authorities have questioned the influence of this funding over the scientific integrity of these organisations.[306]

10 A medicine or a consumer product?

There is a fundamental difference between how medical organisations and consumers view vaping.

The traditional medical model involves going from smoking to complete abstinence as a medical treatment, with professional support and counselling and pharmaceutical aids. Medical treatments are not 'enjoyable'. They are delivered by doctors and are managed by the medicines regulator, the Therapeutic Goods Administration. Success is when smoking and nicotine are completely eliminated.

However, many vapers see it differently. To them, vaping is about replacing one pleasurable consumer behaviour with another far less harmful one. Vaping allows them to continue to enjoy nicotine as well as the many rituals, sensations and social pleasures of smoking. They learn about vaping from other vapers, Facebook groups and online reviewers. Many appreciate the supportive subculture and hobby component of vaping. Success is when smoking is eliminated.

When a large number of Australians tell lawmakers that something is working well for them, they should listen carefully and respectfully. They should acknowledge their lived experience, 'meet them where they are' and empower them to make better decisions about their health.

Vaping nicotine should be regulated by the Australian Competition and Consumer Commission like other consumer products. **No other western country treats nicotine for vaping solely as a medicine and none requires a doctor's prescription.**

21

DEFENDING THE INDEFENSIBLE

Take-home messages

How do you defend an anti-vaping position which is increasingly at odds with the evidence?

- Create fear, doubt, misinformation
- Personal attacks
- Junk science
- Misleading claims from research
- Moral panic
- Use the media to spread misinformation
- Double standards

As it becomes increasingly clear that vaping is far safer than smoking and is helping millions of smokers quit, anti-vaping groups are digging in and desperately trying to defend their position. However, this cannot last forever, and the science will win in the end.

In the meanwhile, how do vaping opponents continue to maintain their opposition when it is no longer supported by the evidence? Sometimes they fight dirty. Here are some examples.

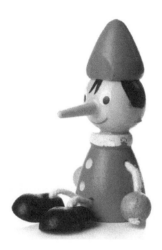

1 Fear, doubt and misinformation

Misinformation about vaping has been spread by respected Australian health and medical authorities and is often reported uncritically in the media, undermining public confidence in vaping.

In the 2010 book *Merchants of Doubt*, Oreskes and Conway explain how the tobacco industry hired a public relations firm to successfully manufacture controversy and uncertainty about the harms from smoking.[307] 'Doubt is our product,' wrote one employee of the Brown & Williamson tobacco company in a 1969 internal memo.[308] The note went on to say that doubt 'is the best means of competing with the "body of fact" and establishing a controversy.'

Today, anti-vaping groups could reasonably be accused of doing the same thing by creating fear and doubt about vaping nicotine. They exaggerate small or theoretical risks and fail to compare them to smoking, minimise the benefits of vaping, use emotive arguments, cherry-pick the evidence and present it in a misleading way.

Vaping has been falsely linked to life-threatening conditions, such as EVALI, Covid-19 and 'popcorn lung'. Misinformation like this is rarely corrected when disproven. The devastating result is that some vapers return to smoking and other smokers are deterred from using vaping to help them quit.

EVALI

It was falsely claimed that a serious lung condition, 'E-cigarette or Vaping-Associated Lung Injury' (EVALI) in the United States in mid-2019 was caused by nicotine vaping.

In August 2019, the cause was found to be vitamin E acetate (VEA), a thickener or 'cutting agent' added to black-market cannabis oils used for vaping in North America.[121] VEA cannot be added to nicotine e-liquids and no cases were linked to nicotine vaping. The outbreak cleared up after VEA was removed from the illicit cannabis supply chain.

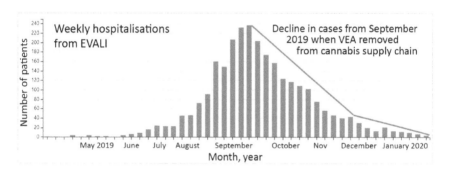

Cases of EVALI declined sharply when the cause was eliminated

However, anti-vaping advocates continued to assert or imply that the condition was caused by nicotine vaping long after that. ATHRA published an exposé in early September 2019.[309] The false claims were not corrected even when the evidence was beyond dispute.[121]

Health authorities were happy to maintain the ambiguity in their publications and websites. A statement by Australia's Chief Medical Officer (CMO) on the Department of Health website in September 2019 claimed that EVALI justified Australia's precautionary approach to nicotine vaping.[310]

Thirty-one leading Australian health professionals sent a critical analysis of this flawed claim to the Chief Medical Officer and state Chief Health Officers asking for a correction in November 2019.[311] However, the misinformation remains unchanged online.

A leading anti-vaping advocate described the EVALI cases as a 'canary in the coalmine' for the health risks of nicotine vaping products in September 2019.[312] In January 2020, the same advocate argued that nicotine vaping caused EVALI because 7% of cases reported that they only vaped nicotine. However, users have an obvious incentive to deny the use of illicit drugs and many deniers were later found to have vaped cannabis.[121]

The result of this misinformation campaign about EVALI was a significant and lasting increase in concerns about the safety of vaping nicotine and reduced uptake.[313,314]

Covid-19

Health authorities and anti-vaping advocates exploited the Covid-19 pandemic to create fear about vaping. Early in the pandemic, they speculated that vaping may increase the risk of catching or transmitting Covid-19 when there was no evidence to support this claim.[315]

For example, VicHealth claimed that 'It's more likely than not that people who smoke or vape have a higher risk of getting coronavirus.'[316]

One study falsely claimed that young people who vaped were five to seven times more likely to test positive for Covid-19.[317] This was promoted by the Australian media [318] but was widely criticised as a flawed conclusion derived from poor research.[319, 320]

Scientific studies have subsequently found no evidence that vaping increases the risk of getting Covid-19[112,321] or transmitting it.[322] However, the damage was already done and the false claims remain uncorrected.

Undermining safety perceptions

Anti-vaping advocates have repeatedly tried to discredit the estimate that vaping is 95% less harmful than smoking, claiming it is not grounded in science, was based on the deliberations of a dubious panel and is therefore invalid.

In fact, the estimate is based on comprehensive and independent reviews of the scientific evidence by Public Health England[55, 84, 97] and the UK Royal College of Physicians[12] and was confirmed in a third scientific review by independent academics.[323]

However, opponents persistently claim that the '95% safer' figure was a 'guesstimate' developed by an expert panel in 2014 convened by Professor David Nutt which assessed the risk of a range of nicotine products.[21, 324,325] This view was widely quoted in the mainstream media[325] and in an article in *The Conversation*.[326]

It was repeated by three anti-vaping Australian academics in a submission to the Australian Parliamentary Inquiry in 2017.[327] In response, Public Health England was forced to confirm that its estimate was based on its 'assessment of the international peer-reviewed evidence relating to the safety of e-cigarettes' and not on the Nutt study.[328]

The Australian newspaper reported, 'Health trio accused of presenting 'factual errors' to the e-cig inquiry.'[329]

The erroneous claim was made yet again in 2020 in a submission by the same academics to the Senate Select Committee on Tobacco Harm Reduction.[330] The lead author of the Public Health England report wrote once again to the committee to correct the record.[331]

Lung Foundation Australia

In an opinion piece in Tasmania's *The Mercury* newspaper on 29 February 2020, the CEO of Lung Foundation Australia (LFA) wrote, 'there is strong, credible evidence that both nicotine and flavoured vaping products are just as harmful, if not more harmful, than conventional cigarettes.'[332]

When the Australian Tobacco Harm Reduction Association (ATHRA) asked the LFA Board in writing to justify or correct this grossly inaccurate claim, no reply was received.[333] Six months later, the LFA released a vaping fact sheet which was riddled with misinformation, as revealed by ATHRA.[334]

Cancer Council Australia and the Heart Foundation

In 2020, Cancer Council Australia and the Heart Foundation circulated a 'fact sheet' to federal members of Parliament which contained multiple significant factual errors. Among other things, it claimed that there is 'no conclusive evidence that e-cigarettes are an effective quit aid,' as well as that 'the claim that e-cigarettes are 95% less harmful than smoking has no basis in science' and that vaping is being used by teenagers, not adult smokers trying to quit. The Australian Tobacco Harm Reduction Association responded to some of the more egregious claims.[335]

Australian Medical Association

Public statements by presidents of the Australian Medical Association have regularly conflicted with the scientific evidence. These have included claims that vaping was 'slightly less harmful than smoking,' in contrast to the overwhelming evidence that it is far safer, and that if you switch to vaping you are still smoking – a curious claim as there is no smoke or combustion involved in vaping.[336] A further statement of concern was that 'There is very clear evidence out there that e-cigarettes are not an effective anti-smoking measure,' when the evidence shows otherwise.[337]

Queensland Health

Australians have the right to assume our governments will give us truthful advice on health matters, based on the latest science. However, Queensland Health (QH) has repeatedly misled the public about vaping and the laws in Queensland.

QH advised the public that it was illegal 'under any circumstances' to import or possess nicotine in Queensland. However, after repeated challenges by ATHRA, QH admitted in July 2018 that it was indeed legal to import nicotine under the Personal Importation Scheme.[338]

QH also claimed in 2019 that it was an offence to bring compounded nicotine liquid (prepared by a compounding pharmacy on prescription) into the state from other parts of Australia, threatening penalties of over $9,000 for 'offenders' who were trying to quit smoking. It was only when challenged again by ATHRA that QH finally admitted that its previous advice was not correct.[339]

The Queensland Health website still provides misleading and unbalanced information about vaping.[340] The online information exaggerates the risks of vaping and omits other important facts and the benefits.

2 Claims of tobacco company funding

A commonly used strategy is to suggest that the public health advocates who favour vaping are tools of Big Tobacco. As a high-profile advocate, this slur has also been directed at me more than once.

On the Alan Jones radio show on 2UE in August 2018, a leading Australian businessman who opposes vaping stated that I am funded by the tobacco industry.[341] This claim is untrue and defamatory. Alan Jones issued a statement on air the next day which correctly stated,

> 'Professor Mendelsohn says much of what Mr Forrest had to say was incorrect, including his claims that vaping is a Big Tobacco conspiracy to hook kids, and that vaping leads to an uptake of smoking in young people. Professor Mendelsohn has also taken exception to Mr Forrest's claim that he's "earned a few bob from big tobacco." He says he's never received any funding or payments from the tobacco industry, and all his lobbying is at his own expense.'[341]

I wrote a letter to Mr Forrest asking for an apology and an opportunity to meet and discuss the evidence. I received a reply suggesting that I should study the science. No apology or correction was made.

In 2020, an article in the *Sydney Morning Herald* claimed that I had 'in the past received funding from tobacco companies.'[342] After I wrote to the editor this was promptly corrected with a statement and an apology. The source of this defamatory comment was not revealed.

In August 2018, the *Sydney Morning Herald* made false claims about the Australian Tobacco Harm Reduction Association (ATHRA), alleging it had received 'secret' industry funding, having been fed this false information by anti-vaping advocates.[343] However, ATHRA rejected this claim. It had previously publicly announced on its website and at an international conference that it had accepted support from the retail vaping industry to help establish the charity. This funding ceased in March 2019. ATHRA has never received funding from the tobacco industry.

3 Junk science

The former editor of the *British Medical Journal*, Richard Smith, estimates that about one in five health studies are either fatally flawed or untrustworthy.[344] This certainly appears to be true in the anti-vaping literature, where numerous 'junk science' studies have been published.

Some researchers start with pre-conceived conclusions and inevitably find the result they are looking for, whether the research supports their claims or not. 'Findings' are often promoted with misleading press releases and get widespread, often uncritical, media coverage.

Other researchers are influenced by the agenda of the funding body. In the US, most research into vaping is funded by the National Institutes of Health which is hostile to vaping. Research outcomes that are not in line with the NIH's agenda may affect future funding opportunities.[345]

The leading anti-vaping researcher and activist, Stanton Glantz from the University of California has been widely criticised for many of his research findings and claims about vaping.[346] One study claimed that vaping was just as likely as smoking to cause heart attacks.[106] This study was flawed but received worldwide media coverage. Further analysis revealed that many of the heart attacks occurred before the subjects began vaping and were more likely to be due to smoking. The study was retracted from the journal in 2020, but by then the damage was already done.[347]

A similar study by Glantz claimed that vaping causes lung disease.[114] This was also widely promoted, for example in *The West Australian* newspaper, 'E-cigarettes a smoking gun for lung disease' (17 December 2019, print edition). Professor John Britton, chairman of the UK Royal College of Physicians Tobacco Advisory Group criticised the findings, writing that the 'conclusion that vaping causes chronic lung disease is fundamentally flawed' as the damage 'would have been present, even though undiagnosed, in many ... cases long before his study began in 2014.'[348] Most of the damage would have been caused by prior smoking. I wrote to the editor of *The West Australian* asking for a correction, but there was no response.

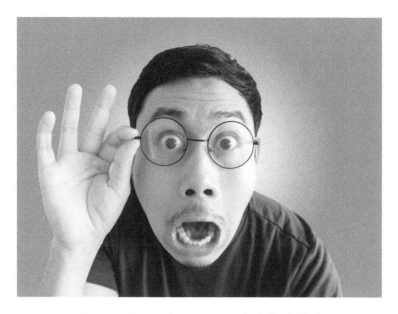

Some vaping junk science simply defies belief

Another widely publicised laboratory study by another author claimed that vaping nicotine produced high levels of formaldehyde, so that the cancer risk from vaping was higher than smoking.[349] However, the study was poorly conducted. A subsequent replication study using the same vaping device found that minimal levels of formaldehyde were emitted.[350]

4 Misleading claims from science

Even when results from scientific studies are technically correct, they are sometimes presented in a misleading way that overstates the risk. Leading vaping advocate Clive Bates lists some of these strategies in a blog, 'The critic's guide to bad vaping science.'[276] Here are five common examples:

Failure to compare harms with smoking

Vaping opponents often raise concerns about small or potential health risks from vaping without comparing the harms to smoking ('relative risk'). This is misleading as vaping is almost exclusively used to replace smoking by current smokers. A minor harm from vaping is justified if it allows switching from the far more harmful behaviour of smoking.

A well-known example was the panic over 'popcorn lung' (bronchiolitis obliterans), a serious disease first detected in popcorn factory workers who were exposed to high doses of diacetyl. A study found small doses of diacetyl in some vapour samples, however no comparison was made with the level of diacetyl in tobacco smoke.[351] It was later revealed that diacetyl levels were 750 times higher in smoke than those found in vapour, and there has never been a case of 'popcorn lung' caused by vaping or smoking.[117]

Exaggerating the risk from trace amounts of chemicals

Numerous studies have created alarm by identifying the presence of a chemical in vapour or e-liquid without measuring the dose.[352] However, this finding is meaningless.[353] There are low doses of chemicals everywhere in the environment, including arsenic in tap water and nineteen known carcinogens in coffee.[354] The important question is whether the dose is sufficient to cause a risk to health. In most cases in vaping studies, the dose did not exceed accepted safety limits, such as those set for occupational or environmental standards and is much lower than in smoke.

Claiming an acute effect causes disease

Some studies find acute effects in the laboratory or in the body from vaping and predict that this will lead to future disease. However, this is not always the case.

For example, Vlachopoulos found that vaping briefly increased the stiffness of blood vessels and raised blood pressure.[355] The author's claim that vaping was as likely as smoking to cause heart disease was breathlessly spread across Australian media outlets. Leading academic Professor Peter Hajek explained that these findings were of no significance. He wrote, 'This is a well-known stimulant effect of nicotine that has little relevance for health. Drinking coffee has the same effect, only greater and longer lasting (as does watching a dramatic football match).'[356]

Confusing 'association' with 'causation'

A common mistake in scientific research is to confuse association with causation.[357] Just because two things are associated (occur together) does not mean one has caused the other. However, anti-vaping researchers have repeatedly made this fundamental error.

Young people who vape are more likely to try smoking later on and some authors claim or imply that this is proof that vaping has caused the smoking.[213] A far more plausible explanation is that young vapers are risk takers. Young people who experiment with vaping are simply more likely to experiment with smoking, drinking, illicit drugs and other risky behaviours as well.[215] If there are cases of causation, they are very rare.

Other studies have claimed that vaping causes heart attacks based on the finding that vapers are more likely to have heart attacks than non-vapers.[358] A more likely explanation is that vapers are former smokers and any increase in heart attack risk was caused by smoking. A careful analysis has shown that there is no evidence that vaping itself increases heart attack risk.[359]

False claims based on animal studies

Harmful effects of vaping found in animal studies are frequently claimed to represent a risk for humans. However, animal studies are a poor guide to outcomes in humans. Animal studies often use unrealistic doses and testing conditions, and animals respond differently to humans. Findings from animals studies do not predict the response in humans in most cases.[113]

Overinterpreting cell studies

In vitro or cell studies in a laboratory often lead to alarming headlines but do not establish a risk of harm in vapers. Studies in test tubes often use excessive doses or continuous exposure, do not replicate real-world use and disregard the role of the body's defences. In most cases the findings do not translate to harm in humans.

5 Moral panic

Vaping critics often use moral panic to create fear about vaping.

Moral panic involves generating public fear about an issue which greatly exceeds the real threat it poses.[360] Moral panic is amplified by the media which needs tantalising news content to generate more clicks and advertising dollars.

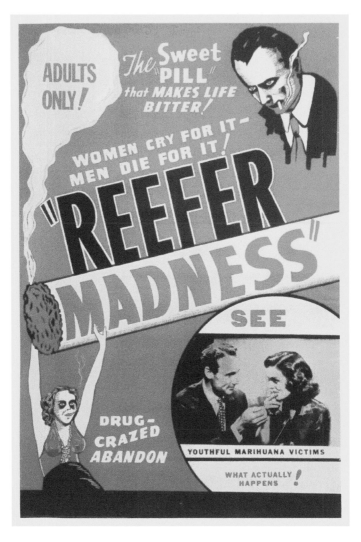

Poster from the movie, Reefer Madness

The moral panic about nicotine is reminiscent of the flagrant propaganda campaign in the 1930s about cannabis, as portrayed in the film *Reefer Madness*. The film was a warning to parents and suggested that 'evil marijuana dealers lurked in public schools, waiting to entice their children into a life of crime and degeneracy.'[361]

The campaign of fear was driven by moral and political motives and used similar strategies to today's anti-vaping campaign: 'protect-the-children' arguments, 'gateway' claims, exaggerations of risks, junk science and selective use of the evidence.

6 Lazy journalism

The media sometimes uncritically spreads misinformation from lay people, doctors and vaping opponents. Several examples from Sydney's *Daily Telegraph* demonstrate this.

On 7 June 2021, the *Daily Telegraph* reported a distraught mother whose son had a seizure and stopped breathing after vaping.[362] She believed that vaping caused the seizure and warned readers that vaping 'is dangerous and can be fatal.' However, there is no evidence that vaping or smoking cause seizures with normal use.[363]

Two anti-vaping advocates provided further inflammatory and misleading comments that sensationalised the story. This misinformation remained unchallenged, as the journalist did not consult a pro-vaping medical expert for verification or balance.

The journalist refused to correct the story and this poor journalism was called out by Alcohol and Other Drugs Media Watch.[364] They stated that 'The paper should have considered its ethical responsibility to this mother and other parents, as well as to expert balance. Demonising vaping undermines the huge potential for vaping nicotine to improve public health in Australia.'

In another story four days later, the *Daily Telegraph* quoted two anti-vaping advocates as saying 'long term use of vapes ... is not better for your health than smoking,' as well as 'switching from smoking to electronic cigarettes has not been shown to reduce proven health harms' and 'the impact [of vaping] on quitting smoking is very weak.' (Vape Craze, A Real Drag, print version, pages 10-11, 11 June 2021)

This blatant misinformation was presented as fact. A pro-vaping expert was not consulted. I wrote to the editor of the *Daily Telegraph* and the journalists responsible, asking for the story to be corrected. I received no reply.

Another article in the *Daily Telegraph* on 31 August 2021 outlined the distressing account of a 19-year-old girl who went to hospital with 'unbearable chest pain' after vaping for 6 months.[365] The Emergency Department doctor diagnosed pleurisy (inflammation of the lining of the lung) due to vaping. It was 'unclear whether she will suffer permanent damage from the incident'.

However, vaping nicotine is not recognised as a cause of pleurisy. There are millions of e-cigarette users globally and there have been no reported cases of pleurisy linked to vaping nicotine. Furthermore, there is no plausible mechanism by which it could occur. Pleurisy is common among healthy young people and is usually due to a viral or bacterial infection.

I wrote to the journalist and editor twice and received no reply. I subsequently prepared a critique of the news story which was published in Alcohol and Other Drugs Media Watch explaining that the report was inaccurate, alarmist and lacked balance.[366]

7 Double standards

Vaping opponents apply double standards to nicotine compared to other drugs or products.

Nicotine classification

The Poisons Standard is Australia's official classification of medicines and poisons that determines their availability and how they are regulated.[367] Nicotine liquid is perversely classified as a dangerous poison or prescription-only product in the Poisons Standard and access is severely restricted. However, nicotine in a far more dangerous form, 'in tobacco prepared and packed for smoking' is specifically excluded from regulation and is freely available as a consumer product.

Long-term research

Anti-vaping advocates demand decades of research into vaping nicotine before they are willing to support it.

A review of submissions to the 2017 parliamentary enquiry into vaping found 'It is common for government agencies and health bodies to assert that unless the safety profile of long-term use of vaping is known, through decades of epidemiological evidence, the current regulatory approach should remain.'[242]

However, this standard is not applied to any other consumer product or medicine. Most medicines are approved after trials of six to twelve months and further harms are monitored in the community.

This hypocrisy was evident in the recent approval of Covid-19 vaccines after trials lasting only months. Suddenly, long-term studies were not needed. However, vaping, with over fifteen years of real-world experience and a large body of scientific research is highly restricted.

Drug harm reduction

Authorities support harm reduction for illicit drugs and alcohol, but not for smoking in spite of a clear commitment to drug harm reduction in Australia's National Drug Strategy (NDS).[286] Harm reduction is one of the three pillars of the NDS to 'Prevent and reduce the adverse health, social and economic consequences associated with alcohol, tobacco and other drug problems.'

Harm reduction strategies are rightly applied to alcohol and other drug use. We accept that people have the right to drink alcohol and we try to reduce the harm, for example by drink-driving laws, responsible alcohol service, liquor licensing and education programs. We accept that some people will use illicit drugs and try to minimise the risks, for example with needle exchange programs, methadone substitution for heroin users and increasingly pill testing and medically supervised injecting rooms.

However, smokers are treated differently. They should just quit and are denied ready access to safer alternatives. Vaping nicotine, the most effective tobacco harm reduction tool, is not supported.

22

HUMAN RIGHTS, AUTONOMY AND SOCIAL JUSTICE

Take-home messages

- Improved access to vaping for adult smokers is supported by
  - The right to optimal health (human rights)
  - National obligations
  - People should be free to act however they wish unless their actions cause harm to someone else (The Harm Principle)
  - The most vulnerable populations are disproportionally affected by smoking, and vaping could help (social justice)
- Australia's laws criminalise honest citizens trying to improve their health

The case for vaping nicotine is also based on the human right to optimal health, the freedom of adults to make their own choices which do no harm to others and the need to protect vulnerable groups who are most affected by smoking.

Human rights

Australia's vaping regulations conflict with the fundamental human right to the best possible health.

The right to health is enshrined in international treaties and conventions. For example, the preamble to the 2006 Constitution of the World Health Organisation states, 'The enjoyment of the highest attainable standard of health is one of the fundamental rights of every human being without distinction of race, religion, political belief, economic or social condition.'[368]

Switching from smoking to a lower-risk nicotine alternative is a clear pathway to improved health for adult smokers who are otherwise unable to quit. Governments have a responsibility to make safer products available and should encourage their use. Instead, Australian law deprives many smokers of this potentially lifesaving opportunity. Smokers have been stigmatised for decade and their rights are given a low priority. A switch from smoking to vaping also protects the rights of bystanders to cleaner air with minimal or no health risk.

Australia's harsh restrictions violate fundamental freedoms and breach its obligations under international treaties such as the Constitution of the World Health Organisation[368] and the Universal Declaration of Human Rights.[369]

Drug use is a health issue not a criminal matter

Australia's unreasonable regulations on vaping nicotine have the perverse effect of criminalising hundreds of thousands of honest Australian citizens who are simply trying to improve their health and are causing no harm to others.

The importation or possession of nicotine e-liquid without a prescription is punishable with severe fines and potential jail terms in Australia.[39, 197] The reality is that most vapers will never have a prescription, making this law a nonsense. More importantly, the laws and the negative messaging discourage smokers from switching to vaping, with profound potential health consequences.

Australia is out of step with international best practice in its approach to nicotine.

- The Global Commission on Drug Policy noted in 2011 that it's time to 'end the criminalization, marginalization and stigmatization of people who use drugs but who do no harm to others.'[370]

- In 2017, the 193 member nations of the United Nations, including Australia, unanimously voted to recognise drug use as a public health issue rather than as a criminal offence.[371] This means taking a compassionate approach which supports and assists drug users.

We are increasingly following this approach in Australia for other drugs but not nicotine.[372] We now need to decriminalise and legalise nicotine e-liquid for vaping to help adult smokers quit, as is the case in all other western democracies.

Criminal charges should be reserved for those involved in illegal manufacture, commercial importation and black-market sales.

The 'Harm Principle'

Australia's paternalistic approach to vaping nicotine is in conflict with the highly respected Harm Principle, developed by the English philosopher John Stuart Mill in 1859.[373]

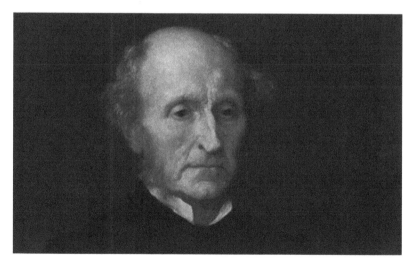

John Stuart Mill. Painting by George Frederic Watts.
National Portrait Gallery, London

The Harm Principle states that people should be free to act however they wish unless their actions cause harm to someone else. Vaping is a 'victimless crime'. Unlike second-hand smoke, there have been no identified health risks to bystanders from vaping according to Public Health England and the UK Royal College of Physicians.[12, 55] Therefore interventions by governments are simply not justified.

Mill states that in a liberal democracy, adults of sound mind should have the freedom and autonomy to make their own lifestyle choices as they know best what is right for themselves whereas governments are often wrong. As with all decisions in life, vapers need to balance the risks and benefits of vaping nicotine and should have the right to choose vaping if it is beneficial to them overall.

Opponents argue that vaping is a risk to young people, but as explained earlier, the evidence does not support this claim. While vaping may lead some young people to smoking, far more are being diverted away from smoking.

Libertarians support vaping as a personal freedom. 'People should decide what they do and don't put in their body. It's not their government's goddamn business' explained Grover Norquist, the founder and President of Americans for Tax Reform.[374]

At the risk of being controversial, we need to also consider the use of recreational nicotine. Nicotine has many positive effects and causes no harm to others. It will likely have a genuine role in the future, alongside caffeine, alcohol, and legalised cannabis.

Social justice

Harsh restrictions on vaping nicotine cause the greatest harm to the most vulnerable members of society and increase health and financial inequalities.

It is unjust that the most vulnerable are disproportionately affected by smoking-related disease and high mortality rates.[375] This is especially true for those on low incomes, people struggling with mental illness or alcohol and drug problems, people with disabilities, the LGBTIQ community, homeless people, Indigenous groups and prisoners.

Smoking is more than twice as common in the poorest members of society than in the most privileged (21% vs 8%).[5] Disadvantaged smokers also smoke more heavily and have lower quit rates.[376] The impoverished, less educated, less tech-savvy and elderly smokers are less able to access nicotine e-liquid through the complex legally mandated pathways.

Smoking is the leading cause of health disparities between the poor and the rich.[377] Traditional tobacco control strategies have had less impact on disadvantaged smokers and health inequalities have increased over time.[378]

There is growing evidence that the uptake of vaping nicotine may be higher in disadvantaged groups.[379-382] The greater use of vaping in these populations could reduce health inequalities.[383-385] Disadvantaged populations 'have many stressors, few resources and a paucity of other rewards in their lives, thus making the transitory 'pleasures' of smoking and the challenges of nicotine withdrawal more salient.[383] For those for whom the 'loss of smoking' is too great, tobacco harm reduction approaches, such as switching to non-smoked nicotine products, should be considered.'[376]

Australia has the highest cigarette prices in the world.[30] This perpetuates poverty and contributes to financial inequalities.[386] Tobacco tax increases are regressive and create financial stress among disadvantaged smokers who can't quit. Vaping is 75-95% cheaper than smoking in Australia and would result in substantial financial savings for the average smoker. Australia's approach to vaping is simultaneously punishing impoverished smokers and is closing a valid escape exit for many who can't otherwise quit.

23

HOW SHOULD VAPING BE REGULATED?

Take-home messages

- It should be easier to access safer vaping products than deadly combustible tobacco
- Nicotine liquid up to 6% should be readily available as a quitting aid for adult smokers with restrictions to minimise access by young people
- Regulation of vaping should be proportionate to the risk which is far less than tobacco products
- Nicotine liquid is a consumer product and should be regulated by the Australian Competition and Consumer Commission
- Enforcement of the ban on the sale of vaping products to young people is a priority
- Other measures to restrict youth vaping include strict age verification for retail and online sales, severe penalties for underage sales, licensing of vape shops and public messaging to frame vaping as a smoking cessation tool for adults
- More comprehensive quality and safety standards are urgently needed
- After-sales monitoring and reporting systems are required
- Accurate public information should be provided to adult smokers

- There is no evidence of risk to bystanders and a nuanced approach to public vaping is needed
- Flavours play an important role in the success of vaping as a quitting aid
- Taxation of vaping products should be kept to a minimum

Regulations for vaping nicotine should be evidence-based, must balance the risks against the benefits, should consider any unintended consequences which may result and be proportionate to risk. Australia's regulations on nicotine vaping fail on all these criteria.

Regulations of vaping should also aim to both reduce youth use and increase access for adult smokers wishing to quit.[205] While both goals are important, Australia's regulations so far have focussed primarily on reducing youth vaping and have largely neglected the substantial opportunity to help adult smokers quit.

New Zealand appears to have found a good balance and its regulations are a suitable model for Australia.[24, 40, 43]

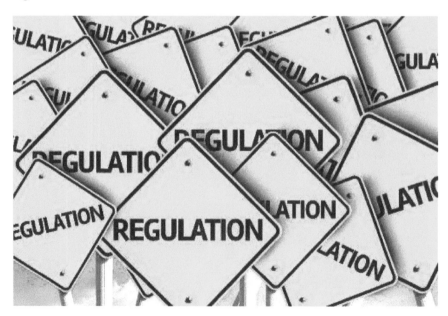

Risk-proportionate regulation

Products are regulated to reduce potential risks to the public. Regulation should be proportionate to risk, so that more dangerous products are controlled more strictly than less harmful ones - the Principle of Proportionality.[387] Perversely, much safer vaping products are regulated more strictly than tobacco products.

Strict controls on smoking are appropriate to reduce the substantial risks that cigarettes pose to public health. However, the risks from vaping nicotine are considerably less. Regulations on vaping should be relaxed to reflect the much lower risk to consumers and to improve access for adult smokers. For the same reason, it would not be appropriate to apply plain packaging rules to vaping products.

Who should regulate vaping?

Vaping products are not medications or poisons in any meaningful sense. They are consumer alternatives to cigarettes with many similar characteristics but dramatically lower risk. They work because they appeal to smokers as alternatives to smoking rather than as medications for treating an illness.

Low concentrations of nicotine liquid (≤6%) are consumer products which compete with another consumer product, combustible cigarettes. They are used almost exclusively as a less harmful substitute for smokers who can't quit smoking or consuming nicotine.

As consumer goods, vaping products should be regulated by the Australian Competition and Consumer Commission (ACCC). The ACCC ensures that consumer products are safe, fit for purpose and comply with all legal requirements under the Competition and Consumer Act 2010.

Currently, nicotine e-liquid is inappropriately regulated as a medicine by Australia's medicine regulator, the Therapeutic Goods Administration (TGA). However, it is not a not medicine or therapeutic good and does not make therapeutic or medicinal claims, such as 'this product will help you quit smoking'. No other western country treats nicotine e-liquid solely as a medicine.

A medicine classification makes vaping products far less accessible and much more expensive for smokers. Users must get a prescription from a doctor and either import liquid nicotine from overseas or find a pharmacy which supplies it. Cigarettes, in contrast, are available from every corner shop and petrol station. It makes no sense to make the less harmful product harder to get than the deadliest consumer product every made.

Specific regulatory issues

Regulation to reduce youth use

Disposable vaping products with nicotine are freely available illegally to underage users from tobacconists, general stores and on social media. Policing and enforcement of black-market sales to youth is almost non-existent and is urgently needed.

Other measures to reduce youth access to vaping include:

- Strict age verification at the time of sale. The minimum age of sale of nicotine e-liquid is currently set by law at 18+ nationally. We need clear guidelines for retailers, with penalties such as loss of licence, as apply to tobacco and alcohol sales.

- Vaping products should only be sold from retail outlets where reliable age verification is available such as vape shops and from retail outlets wherever tobacco is sold.

- Online retailers should verify the age of the purchaser with a third-party age verification service. Commercial services can confirm the age of online buyers and prevent under-age access.

- Verification of age on delivery. This service is currently available and should be mandatory.

- Advertising should be restricted and regulated to prevent appeal to adolescents.

- Public and youth education to frame vaping as a smoking cessation tool or a safer alternative for adult smokers. There should be a clear message that vaping is not for young people or non-smokers.

- Vape shops which sell nicotine e-liquids should be licensed, and admission of under-age shoppers banned. Repeated breaches of this rule should result in substantial penalties and loss of licence.

- Vaping products should not appeal to young people. Products should use generic flavour names only (such as mango) and avoid names that may be especially appealing to young people (such as 'Vampire's Blood'). Packaging should not include cartoons, images and wording which may appeal to young people.[142]

Making it harder for young people to get tobacco cigarettes would reduce smoking and divert young smokers to vaping, a far safer alternative. Strategies to reduce smoking include

- Raising the minimum age of sale of tobacco products from eighteen to twenty-one[142,388]
- Enforcing the minimum age of sale laws for tobacco products
- Reducing the number of tobacco retail outlets

Standards for quality and safety

Basic minimum standards for nicotine e-liquids came into effect in Australia on 1 October 2021, under the Therapeutic Goods (Standard for Nicotine Vaping Products) (TGO110) Order 2021.[118]

Products imported under the Personal Importation Scheme:

- Must not contain added 2,3-pentanedione (acetylpropionyl), acetoin, benzaldehyde, cinnamaldehyde, diacetyl, diethylene glycol, dl-alpha-tocopheryl acetate or ethylene glycol
- Must not contain 'active' ingredients other than nicotine, such as caffeine, THC, stimulants or vitamins

- Should have a maximum nicotine concentration of 100mg/mL
- The nicotine concentration must be within 10% of what is stated
- Compliant labelling and packaging is desirable but not mandatory

Additional requirements apply to products sold through pharmacies including child-resistant packaging, an ingredient list, the nicotine concentration in mg/mL and health warning statements.

Flavours

Some commentators believe that flavours should be restricted due to their appeal to young people.[389] However, while young people like flavours, they are not the primary reason they give for experimenting with vaping in Australia [5] or the US.[225] For example, in the US in 2019, flavours were the third reason given for trying vaping after curiosity and use by a friend or family member.

The uptake of vaping and smoking are much more complex than simply the flavour of the product and include genetic predisposition, smoking by parents and peers, mental health and many other factors.[390] Restricting flavours will not have any effect on these underlying causes.

On the contrary, bans or restrictions on e-liquid flavours can lead to more youth smoking and increased black-market supplies.[391] A ban on flavours in San Francisco was followed by increased smoking by high school students compared to students in other areas, suggesting that vaping flavours were diverting young people from smoking (see figure below).[392] When US manufacturer JUUL removed its fruit- and sweet-flavoured products due to concerns about youth uptake, users simply switched to mint, menthol and tobacco flavours, with no overall reduction in use.[393]

However, flavours make vaping more appealing as an alternative for adult smokers.[189] Flavours encourage the uptake of vaping by current smokers, reduce the likelihood of relapse[189] and are associated with higher quit rates compared to non-flavoured or tobacco flavoured e-liquids.[187, 224]

In a survey of 35,000 nicotine users in the European Union, '71% of vapers would look for alternative sources to the legal market' if there was a flavour ban.[394] In another survey of 550 young adult vapers in the US, 39% said they would switch to smoking if flavours were restricted to tobacco-only.[395]

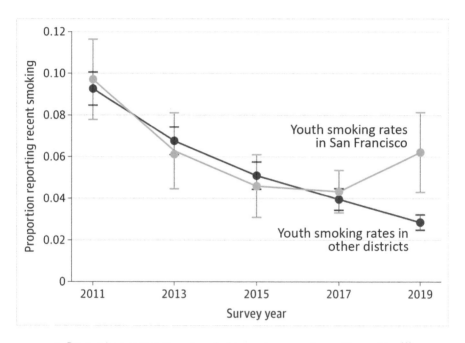

A flavour ban in San Francisco led to an increase in youth smoking[392]

Nicotine gum is available in Australia in fruit, mint, spearmint and icy mint flavours and research shows that flavoured nicotine gum enhances its appeal and improves compliance.[396]

Retail sale

Vaping products with nicotine should be at least as accessible as cigarettes and sold wherever age-of-sale laws can be enforced. This should include vape shops, tobacconists, pharmacies and general stores.

In Australia, nicotine liquid can only be purchased from pharmacies, with a doctor's prescription. In the UK, vape shops can sell nicotine vaping products and some have been set up in National Health Service hospitals.[397]

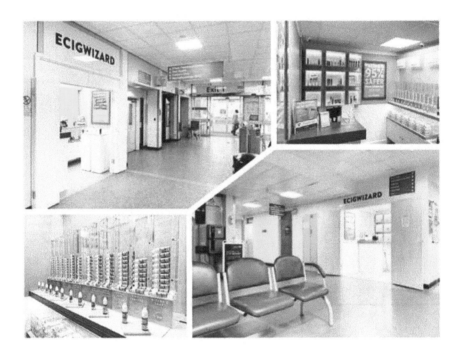

Vape shop in an NHS hospital in the UK (permission from Ecigwizard)

Clear public health messaging

People have a right to accurate health information.[240] This should inform adult smokers of the potential benefits and risks of vaping and reinforce the message that vaping is not for young people or non-smokers. However, the risks should not be exaggerated nor should the benefits be overstated.

Accurate public health messaging could include:

- Vaping is not risk-free but is far less harmful than smoking

- Vaping is an effective smoking cessation tool for adult smokers who are unable to quit with the available treatments and would otherwise continue to smoke

- Vaping is not for young people or non-smokers
- Completely quitting smoking gives the best health outcomes
- Vapers should try to quit vaping but only if they are able to avoid relapsing to smoking
- There is no evidence so far that second-hand vapour is harmful
- Vapers should vape considerately and respect the rights of bystanders to breathe fresh air

The UK Royal College of Physicians recommends:[142]

- Mass media campaigns to support the use of vaping as a quitting aid or substitute for smoking to correct false perceptions about the safety of vaping compared with cigarettes.

- 'Health warnings on e-cigarette packs include a statement that e-cigarette vapour is likely to be substantially less harmful than tobacco smoke.'

Public vaping

There is no evidence that vaping nicotine poses a health risk to bystanders and a blanket ban in public places is not justified on public health grounds. Hazardous agents are present at such low concentrations in exhaled vapour that they pose no meaningful risk to bystanders.[398]

Bans on public vaping send the misleading message that vaping is just as harmful as smoking. Allowing vaping in smoke-free areas makes vaping more appealing and provides an added incentive to switch to the less harmful product. Vapers who have switched from smoking may be more likely to relapse if they are forced into smoking areas with smokers.

Exposure to second-hand vapour is a nuisance or etiquette issue which can be managed by public education and appropriate signage. Property owners and managers should be able to make their own decisions about vaping for staff, clients or customers on their premises, as occurs in the UK.[399] For example, the Royal Australian and New Zealand College of Psychiatrists recommends allowing vaping in smoke-free mental health facilities.[400]

There is no justification for outdoor vaping bans. The risk of exposure outside is even lower and 'it seems unlikely that the use of e-cigarettes would have a measurable impact on outdoor air quality.'[142]

Because of the value of vaping in supporting abstinence, the UK Royal College of Physicians recommends allowing vaping in some public and indoor premises and that 'smoke-free policies should not automatically be extended to include non-tobacco nicotine use.'[142]

Advertising

The current ban on advertising vaping products protects the market domination by cigarettes.

Carefully regulated advertising of vaping products could raise awareness of vaping as a quitting aid. Smokers exposed to television advertisements for vaping are more likely to quit smoking.[401]

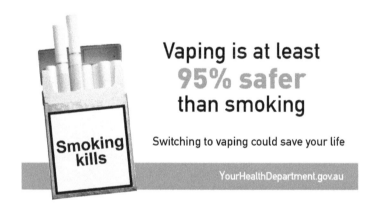

Advertising should target switching by adult smokers

Advertising should focus on a switching theme – as a safer substitute for adult smokers who have been unable to quit – and should not appeal to youth, as outlined in the UK code of non-broadcast advertising.[402] Strict controls should be applied to the content and placement of advertisements as is the case for alcohol advertising.

Taxation

A number of studies have shown that price rises on vaping products increase smoking and reduce vaping in both adults[403-405] and teenagers[406] confirming that vaping products are substitutes for smoking.

Taxation on vaping products should be proportionate to their harm compared to tobacco.[142] The UK Royal College of Physicians recommends a tax of 5% to make 'reduced harm alternatives [to smoking] much more affordable' to encourage switching.[142]

High taxes on vaping products would also increase the appeal of cheaper black-market products. In the EU Nicotine Users Survey in 2020, more than 60% of vapers said they would look for alternative untaxed sources if a high excise was applied to e-liquid.[394]

Low taxes are especially important for low-income and disadvantaged groups who have the highest smoking rates and are most impacted by the financial stress from smoking.

Monitoring and recall

A system is needed to report side-effects and safety concerns from vaping products. For example, the UK has established a 'Yellow Card' reporting system for consumers and healthcare professionals.[407]

A procedure for recalling unsafe or non-complaint goods is also required.

Further information

The Australian Tobacco Harm Reduction Association has prepared a Discussion Paper on Regulation of Nicotine E-Liquids for Vaping in Australia, which provides further detail.[408]

24

THE FUTURE OF VAPING IN AUSTRALIA

Take-home messages

- Political pressure from individuals, organisations and the general public is the key to change
- Change can be accelerated by
  - Advocacy by vapers and advocacy groups
  - Public education to correct misperceptions and engage public support
  - Legal challenges
  - Responsible, accurate and balanced reporting by media outlets
  - The retirement of leading anti-vaping figures
  - Education and training of doctors
- Change in the entrenched anti-vaping views of Australian medical organisations is unlikely in the short-medium term, despite the growing and compelling evidence

The debate on vaping nicotine in Australia is at a stalemate. Federal and state governments, peak health organisations, health charities and most medical associations remain opposed. These groups dominate the narrative and the media, promoting a 'precautionary', wait-and-see approach.

Australia's regulations on vaping are harming public health, however they could get a lot worse. Anti-vaping organisations are campaigning for flavour bans, limits on nicotine concentration, nicotine import bans and higher taxation which would further undermine the appeal and effectiveness of vaping. These misguided changes are currently being introduced in Canada.[409]

Harm reduction strategies[204] and disruptive technologies[301] are relentlessly opposed in the short-term but triumph in the long-term, and vaping will be no different. As community pressure builds and the evidence becomes undeniable, a tipping point will be reached. Vaping nicotine will eventually become a mainstream quitting aid and perhaps even accepted as an adult recreational activity.

However, there needs to be more urgency. Advocacy and political pressure can, and must, accelerate this process. While we wait for change, over 21,000 Australians will continue to die prematurely every year from smoking. Vaping nicotine could prevent many of these deaths.

1 Social movements, advocacy and political pressure

'A social movement is a loosely organized effort by a large group of people to achieve a particular goal, typically a social or political one. This may be to carry out, resist or undo a social change. It is a type of group action and may involve individuals, organizations or both.'[410]

Social movements have a long history of creating change in Australia. Examples include same-sex marriage, women's rights, the climate movement and, more recently, the MeToo movement and assisted dying.

Ultimately, the decision to relax the laws on vaping nicotine is political and will be made in the Federal Parliament. However, State and Territory Parliaments can also make laws to change the regulations in their own jurisdictions.

There are now well over 500,000 vapers in Australia and the number is increasing rapidly. If vapers, their friends and families speak out, vaping will have the clout needed to trigger political change before long.

There are many MPs in Canberra who support vaping. However, political parties will only tackle a controversial policy when a critical mass of public support is reached and the political risk of changing policy is considered acceptable. Active campaigning in marginal seats is a widely used strategy for political pressure and should be introduced for vaping.

The health minister also needs political cover from the community and supportive health groups to make a major policy change which will be opposed by many influential organisations.

Community outrage led to a policy change on vaping in June 2020. The minister for health suddenly announced a complete ban on importing nicotine liquid to begin on 1 July. This threat galvanised the vaping community.[411]

Vapers contacted their MPs, a petition against the changes collected 72,000 signatures in a couple of days, vapers and advocates flooded social and mainstream media. Twenty-eight federal coalition backbenchers wrote to the prime minister condemning the changes. The health minister was forced to back down and announced on 26 June 2020 that the plan would be delayed. Later it was cancelled altogether.

In May 2021, the Therapeutic Goods Administration announced that nicotine e-liquid could now be sold in Australian chemists and online pharmacies.[23] Although this scheme requires a doctor's prescription, it was another concession by the minister in response to the pressure from vaping advocates.

Individual advocacy

The life-changing stories of individual vapers are powerful and compelling and are the key to change. Vapers should share their personal experience with anyone who will listen. Tell your friends, workmates and other smokers. Share your story on social media. Contact your local radio station or the mainstream media when the opportunity arises. Correct the misinformation about vaping with your lived experience, whenever you get the opportunity.

Writing to your federal and state members of parliament is essential for every vaper. Arrange an appointment and take your vaping friends with you. Explain how vaping has changed your lives for the better.

Vapers could play a valuable role in educating their doctors. If vaping has helped you quit smoking, tell your doctor. Personal stories can cut through when the evidence does not. Explain how switching to vaping has improved your health and wellbeing and the health and budget of your family.

Some GPs are not aware that the Royal Australian College of General Practitioners has acknowledged a role for nicotine vaping in its most recent smoking cessation guidelines and you could mention this.[4]

In the UK, vapers played a major role in the early acceptance and uptake of vaping. Vapers told their stories at conferences and engaged with, and educated, key stakeholders.

A small number of vapers have been active in advocacy in Australia, but the vast majority have stayed below the radar. The reasons for this include the illegal nature of vaping nicotine (without a nicotine prescription) and the stigma associated with smoking and vaping. Many vapers get their supplies easily from overseas and do not see the need for change.

However, vapers also need to advocate for the three million smokers in Australia who could benefit from vaping nicotine. Finding information and switching to vaping is a challenging process in the current environment. Accessing supplies from overseas is impossible for many disadvantaged and vulnerable smokers. Advocacy will improve access for current smokers and facilitate switching.

Advocacy organisations

Advocacy organisations to represent vapers and the vaping industry are urgently needed in Australia. Anti-vaping lobby groups are well funded and are in regular contact with parliamentarians in Canberra. MPs need to also hear the other side of the vaping story.

A new Australian advocacy group was being formed at the time of writing to advocate for all safer nicotine products including vaping nicotine, heated tobacco products and oral nicotine products such as snus and nicotine pouches. All vapers are encouraged to become members when it is fully registered.

Similar vaper advocacy groups are successfully operating in many other countries, such as AVCA in New Zealand, NNA in the UK, CASAA in the US and CAPHRA in the Asia Pacific region.

Many fall under the umbrella of the International Network of Nicotine Consumer Organisations (www.innco.org) but some are independent.

Australia also urgently needs an effective vape industry lobbying group. The Australian Retail Vaping Industry Association (ARVIA) was launched in November 2019 under the Australian Retailers Association but was disbanded about a year later. Vape shops are currently represented under the umbrella of the National Retail Association but very little is being done.

Strong vape industry organisations exist in other countries, such as the Independent British Vape Trade Association (www.ibvta.org.au) and the Vape Industry Association (www.ukvia.co.uk) in the UK and the Vapor Technology Association (www.vaportechnology.org) and American Vapor Manufacturers Association (www.theavm.org) in the US.

There are two other organisations in Australia that support and advocate for vaping and tobacco harm reduction.

- The Australian Tobacco Harm Reduction Association is a health promotion charity established by doctors to raise awareness of safer nicotine products such as vaping and to encourage change in public policy. Their focus is on helping smokers quit and improving public health. (www.athra.org.au)

- Legalise Vaping Australia is part of the Australian Taxpayers' Alliance. It 'is dedicated to campaigning for the legalisation and risk proportionate regulation of vaping and e-cigarettes across Australia.' (www.legalisevaping.com.au)

2 Public education and the media

The general public is seriously misinformed about vaping. Most people incorrectly think vaping nicotine is just as harmful as, if not more harmful than, smoking. This is the result of a fear and misinformation campaign by vaping critics, amplified by alarmist media reports. This has to change. The public should be given accurate and honest information about vaping to raise awareness of its true value to public health.

The New Zealand Ministry of Health has established *The Facts of Vaping* website (www.vapingfacts.health.nz) which presents accurate information about vaping and encourages its uptake by adult smokers who are unable to quit.[24] A similar online government resource is needed for Australian smokers.

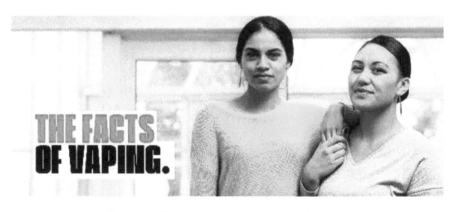

The Facts of Vaping, www.vapingfacts.health.nz

While there are some high-quality media reports on vaping, too many articles are inaccurate and sensational and discourage smokers from switching. This will ultimately lead to more death and disease from smoking.

Media outlets should take the lead by ensuring more responsible and balanced reporting. Journalists have an ethical obligation to present scientific evidence fairly. Here are some tips from the Australian Science Media Centre, *Sydney Morning Herald guidelines* and Health News Review:

- Avoid alarmist and sensational headlines

- Avoid focusing just on negative news; tell your audience about good news as well

- Provide balanced coverage. Seek independent comments from others with expertise in the field

- Put risk into perspective by comparing it to smoking or some other benchmark; absolute numbers provide readers with more information to determine the true size of the benefit

- Treat research on animals and cells with great caution, making it clear that the results may not translate to humans

- Distinguish between association and causation

- Avoid uncritical publication of vaping science based on a press release; read and analyse the research study

- Be wary of small studies and single-anecdote news stories

3 Legal action

There are several potential legal pathways to challenge Australia's unjust and harmful laws on vaping nicotine. These include under 'delegated legislation', civil liberties, human rights and restraint of trade.

Legal action can be costly but has been successful in several western countries. Courts have ruled that harsh restrictions on vaping, Swedish snus and heated tobacco products are an overreach by governments. There are opportunities for similar challenges in Australia.

In 2018, Philip Morris New Zealand took the Ministry of Health to court to challenge the ban on heated tobacco products (HTPs). The District Court ruled that a ban was not consistent with the Smoke-Free Environments Act, as HTPs were less harmful than smoking and would improve the health of smokers.[412] The ruling allowed HTPs as well as nicotine liquid for vaping to be legally sold to adults as consumer products in New Zealand.

In 2019, the Quebec Vaping Association challenged Quebec's laws that treated vaping like smoking. The Quebec Superior Court ruled that the restrictions on vaping violated the fundamental rights of smokers by denying them access to a safer alternative.[413]

In 2019, the Swiss Federal Supreme Court used similar reasoning to overturn the ban on the sale of Swedish snus, a low-risk non-combustible tobacco product which replaces smoking.[414]

4 Generational change

Leading figures in the anti-vaping movement are personally invested in their opposition to vaping and will not change their positions no matter how much evidence is produced. Some individuals have considerable influence over vaping policy and establishment views. When key leaders retire, the next generation may be more open to change and more supportive of vaping.

The Nobel prize winning physicist Max Planck made the following depressing observation,

> 'a new scientific truth does not triumph by convincing its opponents and making them see the light but rather because its opponents eventually die, and a new generation grows up that is familiar with it.'[415]

5 Doctors

The medical profession is conservative and tends to follow advice from official government and medical sources. Some doctors support vaping, but most are sceptical and poorly informed. The Australian Medical Association (AMA) remains opposed to vaping and is highly vocal.

However, there has been some progress with the professional associations or 'Colleges'. Psychiatrists strongly endorsed vaping in 2018.[400] The College of GPs recognised vaping as a legitimate second-line quitting aid in 2020.[4] Physicians showed some softening in their position in 2020.[416]

Doctors also need formal education on vaping, but this is unlikely to occur to any extent. Doctors receive very little training in smoking cessation, and most is sponsored by the pharmaceutical industry to promote stop-smoking medications. Unlike the United Kingdom which has a National Centre for Smoking Cessation and Training (www.ncsct.co.uk), Australia does not have an organisation dedicated to training health professionals on smoking cessation.

Training could be provided by the Royal Australian College of General Practitioners or independent training organisations with federal funding or vape industry support. If training is provided, it should cover the information in Parts 1 and 2 of this book, so doctors can advise and support smokers to switch to vaping if appropriate. Teaching should always include the 'real experts' – former smokers who have quit with vaping who can relate their lived experience.

6 Health and medical organisations

I have been actively involved in vaping advocacy since 2015 and have seen very little change in the views of Australia's leading health and medical organisations.

Dr Alex Wodak and I have met with and written to many of them, including the minister for health, the National Health and Medical Research Council, the Therapeutic Goods Administration, the Cancer Council, Heart Foundation Australia, Lung Foundation Australia and the Thoracic Society. However, they have shown no sign of softening their attitudes, even as the evidence in favour of vaping continues to build. If anything, they have become more entrenched in their anti-vaping view and increasingly unwilling to debate or discuss the issues.

Their positions on vaping reflect neither the best available scientific evidence nor the overseas experience. Their views should not be accepted uncritically, as if they are unquestionable authorities on this subject.

These organisations are respected and influential in health policy in Australia. As the scientific evidence accumulates and their opposition to vaping become increasingly untenable, they risk losing community trust and respect.

In an ideal world, pro- and anti-vaping organisations would objectively examine the evidence together, discuss their own biases, acknowledge the unintended consequences of their policies and negotiate trade-offs, finally agreeing on a workable compromise that is best for public health. In my view, this is unlikely in the short term.

Rather than trying to persuade vaping opponents, the limited time and resources of pro-vaping advocates are better spent on educating their friends, families, the public, doctors and politicians.

Conclusion

The future of vaping depends on your efforts. If you are a vaper, do it for yourself. If a loved one smokes, do it for them. Do it for the three million smokers and future generations who should have access to lifesaving vaping products.

Progress requires a mass social movement across the whole community. Individual vapers and their supporters need to tell their stories. All vapers should join the Australian Vaping Advocacy Group and an active industry representative group is urgently needed. The public needs to be educated about the evidence for vaping and its potential for improving public health. Responsible, balanced and accurate reporting by the media is vital. Members of parliament need to hear the lived experiences of their constituents.

A change in policy will follow once there is sufficient public support and political pressure. It always does, but the sooner the better.

The lives and wellbeing of hundreds of thousands of Australian smokers depend on it.

APPENDIX

GLOSSARY

18650
The most common size of lithium-ion battery used for vaping. It is 18mm high and 65mm long.

510
The most common style of 'threading' for vaping devices. Tanks and batteries that are both 510-threaded can be screwed together.

Amps (amperes)
The unit of electrical current. The amp reading on a vaping device refers to how much current is passing through the circuit. According to Ohm's law, the higher the voltage and the lower the resistance of the coil, the more current will go through the coil. There are 1000 milliamps to one amp.

Atomiser
The component that heats the e-liquid into an aerosol. It is located in the tank of e-liquid and consists of a heating coil, a wick and a case or housing. In vaping, the terms atomiser and coil are used interchangeably although strictly the coil is part of the atomiser.

Box mod
An advanced, box-shaped vaping device which can be modified by the user. You can adjust the power output, temperature level, airflow and other settings which are displayed on digital screen. Box mods are larger and more powerful than other vaping devices.

Bricks-and-mortar store
A physical store where you can buy vaping devices, nicotine-free liquids and accessories and get expert advice from staff.

Carcinogen
A substance known to cause cancer.

Cartomiser
A cartridge for a cigalike made of a heating coil and liquid vapour and filled with an absorbent material. Disposable and refillable versions are available.

Chipset
A tiny, printed circuit board (PCB) which is the brains of a vaporiser. The chipset controls the operations of the vape, keeping it operating safely and allowing you to customise settings, such as power and temperature.

Cigalike
A low-powered vaping device which has the look and feel of a traditional cigarette. Cigalikes have no buttons or controls and are easy to use. They are either disposable or rechargeable.

Clearomiser
The clear, transparent tanks used in vape pens and box mods. Clearomisers contain the e-liquid, coil and wick and allows you to see how much liquid you have left.

Cloud(s)
The vapour that is exhaled when vaping.

Cloud chasing
Refers to making large clouds when you vape. Those who engage in cloud chasing are called 'cloud chasers.'

Coil
The heating element that vaporises the e-liquid when electricity from the battery passes through it.

Compounding pharmacy
A specialty pharmacy that makes a medication prescribed by a doctor for a specific patient from the basic ingredients.

Diacetyl
A harmful compound used to give a buttery flavour which has been found in some e-juices, although at levels far below those found in cigarette smoke. It is now banned in Australia.

Direct-to-lung (DTL)
A style of inhalation used for vaping. It involves taking a draw of vapour directly into the lungs in one movement, like taking a deep breath before diving into the water. DTL vaping produce large clouds and greater flavour.

Doubler
A half-filled bottle of nicotine-free e-juice at twice the flavour concentration. To make nicotine e-liquid, you add the same volume of unflavoured nicotine at double the strength you vape to get the final nicotine concentration you want.

Dry puff or dry hit
A dry puff occurs from heating a dry wick. The result is burning the coil and wick, releasing a foul-smelling discharge that contains higher levels of toxins. It can also occur when using a power setting that is too high for your coil, chain vaping (taking many puffs in a row) or not priming (saturating) a new coil before using it. It is a good idea to refill your tank or pod when it gets to around a third full.

DIY mixing
Making your own customised e-liquid by mixing the individual ingredients yourself. DIY is cheaper than using pre-mixed e-liquids and many enjoy it as a hobby. DIY mixing requires purchasing high concentrations of nicotine and is not generally recommended for beginners.

Dripping

A method of dripping drops of e-liquid directly onto the heating coil instead of feeding e-liquid from a tank. Claimed to produce better flavour and cloud production but can generate more harmful chemicals.

Drip tip

The mouthpiece that fits into the top of the vaping device. Drip tips are made from a variety of different materials and come in many shapes and sizes.

E-liquid

The liquid solution used in vaping devices. E-liquid or e-juice contains four ingredients: nicotine (optional), flavourings, propylene glycol (PG) and vegetable glycerine (VG).

ENDS

Electronic Nicotine Delivery Systems. Another term for electronic cigarettes.

EVALI

Electronic-cigarette or Vaping product use–Associated Lung Injury (EVALI) is a serious lung condition in people who had recently vaped in the US in 2019. This condition has now been clearly linked to black-market cannabis oils contaminated with Vitamin E Acetate, purchased from street dealers. No cases were linked to commercial nicotine vaping products.

Flavouring

Flavourings are an integral part of the appeal of vaping. Smokers typically begin with tobacco flavour, but most progress to fruit, dessert, food, mint or beverage flavours over time. Most of the flavouring chemicals are food flavourings and are safe to swallow, but less is known about their safety for inhalation.

Freebase nicotine

Freebase nicotine is mainly used in low concentrations in high wattage devices, such as box mods and vape pens. It provides the familiar 'throat hit' (the sensation at the back of the throat) which is part of the smoking experience. At high concentrations, freebase nicotine can be harsh and irritating to the throat. Typical concentrations range from 6-24mg/mL. See also nicotine salt.

Kanthal wire
A popular metal alloy used for making coils. It is made from iron, chromium and aluminium.

Lithium-ion battery
The most popular type of battery used for vaping devices. The battery supplies electricity to heat the coil and convert the e-liquid into a vapour. Also widely used in mobile phones, laptop computers and even electric cars.

mAh
The capacity of the battery is measured in mAh (milliamp hours) and tells you how long it can last on a single charge. Most batteries are in the range of 300-2500 mAh.

Mechanical mod
A vaping device which contains no safety features such as short circuit protection, overcharge protection or overheat protection. There is a much greater safety risk of battery malfunction, burnt coils and overheating. 'Mech mods' are not recommended for novice vapers.

Mesh coil
One kind of heating coil, essentially a strip of metal with holes punched in it. Mesh coils heat more quickly and produce more flavour.

Mods
An advanced vaping device which can be modified in various ways. For example, power and temperature can be adjusted and coils, tanks and batteries can be replaced.

Mouth-to-lung (MTL)
A two-stage inhalation style used initially by most beginner vapers. MTL is similar to smoking and helps vapers make the transition away from smoking. You first draw the vapour into your mouth for several

seconds and then inhale into the lungs as a second step. MTL is a more discreet vaping style which produces smaller clouds.

Nichrome
A popular metal alloy used for making coils. It is made from chromium and nickel.

Nicotine
The main chemical causing dependence in tobacco smoke and vapour. In the low concentrations used in smoking and vaping it is relatively benign and also has positive effects, such as improved concentration and weight control.

Nicotine salt
A form of nicotine made by adding an acid (such as benzoic, lactic or salicylic acid) to freebase nicotine. Nicotine salts are smoother to inhale and allow you to use higher doses with less throat irritation. Nicotine salts are also absorbed more quickly than freebase nicotine and have a more rapid effect like the nicotine from smoking.

Nicotine shot
Small bottles of freebase nicotine or nicotine salt (usually 10-20 mL) in various concentrations. The full bottle is added to a partly filled bottle of flavoured e-liquid (a 'shortfill' bottle) to make flavoured nicotine e-liquid.

Ohm
The standard unit of electrical resistance represented by the symbol Ω. A coil with low resistance heats more quickly and are used to produce larger vapour clouds.

Ohm's Law
Voltage = Current x Resistance. A formula used to calculate Voltage (watts), coil Resistance (ohms) and current (amps) for more advanced users. By knowing any two of the three values, you can calculate the third.

Pods
A cartridge containing a coil, wick and e-liquid which can be connected to and removed from a vape battery.

Pod vape
A compact vaporiser consisting of a pod of nicotine salt and a vape battery. Some models use prefilled pods and others can be refilled by the user.

Popcorn lung
'Popcorn lung' (bronchiolitis obliterans) is a serious, but rare lung disease first detected in popcorn factory workers caused by high levels of diacetyl, a flavouring agent. It has been suggested that low doses of diacetyl from vaping may cause popcorn lung, but there has never been a case of bronchiolitis obliterans due to vaping.

Premixed e-liquid
Premixed e-liquid is purchased ready to vape and contains nicotine (optional), flavouring, propylene glycol and vegetable glycerine. It is available in bottles or pods.

Priming
The process of soaking your new coil prior to use. This reduces the chances of dry burn and burnt-out coils.

Propylene glycol (PG)
Propylene glycol (propane-1,2 diol) is a clear, tasteless liquid found in almost all e-liquids. PG helps to create the familiar 'throat hit' that smokers are used to and helps to carry the flavouring in the e-liquid. PG is generally regarded as safe but there is limited experience with long term inhalation.

Rebuildable dripping atomiser
An atomiser in which you make your own coils and wicks and drip e-liquid directly onto the coil before vaping. There is no tank of e-liquid.

Rebuildable tank atomiser
Vaping tanks in which you use own home-made coils and wicks. Once you add e-liquid to the tank they work like regular vaping tanks.

Resistance
The degree to which the coil opposes electrical current through it and is measured in ohms. Low-resistance coils are used with high powered devices for making larger clouds. Higher resistance coils are better for mouth-to-lung vaping and smaller clouds.

Shortfill
A bottle of flavoured nicotine-free liquid which is only partly filled. 'Nicotine shots' are added to make flavoured nicotine e-liquid.

Snus
Swedish snus is a moist, finely ground tobacco product usually supplied in sachets like small teabags which are placed under the upper lip. Nicotine from snus is slowly absorbed through the lining of the mouth. Snus is used as a quitting aid or as a long-term safer source of nicotine.

Squonk

A squonk mod (squonker) is a type of advanced, unregulated mod – i.e., it does not have wiring, circuitry, a computer chip or a board. The mod contains a plastic or silicone bottle of e-liquid which can be squeezed to force e-liquid directly onto the atomiser. Squonks are not for beginners.

Stealth vaping
Vaping discreetly to avoid drawing attention to your vaping.

Sub-ohm vaping
Vaping with a low coil resistance of < 1 ohm, which creates larger clouds and more intense flavour. Sub-ohm vaping is usually done with a high-powered device and low nicotine concentrations, typically 3-6mg/mL.

Steeping
The process of allowing time for newly made e-liquid mixtures to blend and settle before using them. This can take days or weeks.

Throat hit
The sensation felt in the back of the throat when inhaling from a cigarette mostly caused by nicotine. A good throat hit from vaping is important for some smokers to mimic the smoking experience, making the transition from smoking to vaping easier.

Tobacco Harm Reduction
A strategy for reducing the harm from smoking by switching to a safer nicotine product rather than aiming for complete abstinence from nicotine. It is for smokers who cannot or will not quit and would otherwise continue to smoke.

Unregulated mods
Mods that do not have wiring, circuitry or a chipset and are not as safe as regulated devices. They should only be used by experienced users who are fully informed on their correct use.

Vape pens
Cylindrical vaporisers shaped like a pen. They consist of a battery compartment and a refillable tank.

Vaping
The act of inhaling vapour from an electronic vaporiser.

Variable wattage
Advanced vaporisers have variable wattage so that you can adjust the power output of the device. This can affect the vapour production and flavour and allows you to customise your vaping experience.

Vegetable glycerine
A clear, viscous ingredient in e-liquid which increases vapour production. It is generally regarded as very safe although there is limited information on long-term inhalation.

Wattage
A watt is the unit of power and indicates how much power can be produced for the device. More power is needed for direct-to-lung vaping and larger clouds.

Wick

An absorbent material usually made from organic cotton that draws e-liquid from a reservoir to the coil so that it can be vaporised. Other materials used for wicking include silica, rayon and stainless steel.

ADDITIONAL RESOURCES

Online forums

Vaping in Australia
An Australian forum for sharing information on vaping and supporting new vapers.
https://vapinginaustralia.com/

Vapers Down Under
A popular Reddit discussion and support group for Australian vapers with 13,000 members.
https://www.reddit.com/r/aussievapers/

E-cigarette Forum
The world's largest vaping website with discussion forums, product information and blogs.
https://www.e-cigarette-forum.com/

Facebook groups

Vape Fam Australia
A popular Australian page, very friendly and helpful for new users.
https://www.facebook.com/groups/2970172996629644

Muffs-A-Puffin
Supportive group for women who love to vape and share experiences and stories about vaping.
https://www.facebook.com/groups/2180340605617746/

DIY Downunder 18+

A group dedicated to the do-it-yourself e-liquid mixing.

https://www.facebook.com/groups/diydownunder/

Pods Australia

An Australasian Facebook group for pod users to meet online and share information about pod vapes.

https://www.facebook.com/groups/PodVapersAustralia

Online resources

Australian Tobacco Harm Reduction Association (ATHRA)

www.athra.org.au

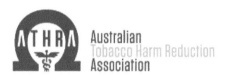

ATHRA is an independent Australian health promotion charity established by doctors to provide accurate information about vaping for adult smokers who are unable to quit with other methods. ATHRA is funded by tax-deductible donations from the public and does not accept funding from the vaping or tobacco industries.

The ATHRA website has a wide range of evidence-based information on vaping. It also covers smoking and its health effects and evidence-based advice on traditional quitting methods. It has a special section for health professionals who want to know more about vaping and nicotine prescribing.

New Zealand Ministry of Health

https://vapingfacts.health.nz/ and https://quitstrong.nz/switch-vaping

UK National Health Service

https://www.nhs.uk/smokefree/

Vaping 360

A reputable commercial site with an excellent blog, product reviews and good advice on a wide range of vaping topics.
https://vaping360.com/

E-cigarette Academy

A UK-based commercial site with excellent articles for beginners and advanced users. https://www.ecigarettedirect.co.uk/ashtray-blog/category/ecigarette-academy

'Mooch'

Information about batteries and electronics from a leading expert.
https://facebook.com/batterymooch

Australian reviewers

A number of vaping experts produce regular YouTube videos about vaping news, reviews of new devices and advocacy. These are entertaining and informative.

Legion Vapes (Steve)
https://www.youtube.com/legionvapes

The Vaping Bogan (Sam)
https://www.youtube.com/TheVapingBogan
Language alert! Not for sensitive viewers.

Friday Vape Club (Squidly)
https://www.youtube.com/FridayVapeClub

The Aussie Vape Show
https://www.facebook.com/The-Aussie-Vape-Show
A weekly live panel show.

International reviewers

GrimmGreen
Nick is the leading international vaping reviewer and commentator with over 390,000 subscribers.
https://www.youtube.com/GrimmGreen

Phil Busardo
https://www.youtube.com/pbusardo

Rip Trippers
https://www.youtube.com/RipTrippers

Vic Mullin
https://www.youtube.com/VapingWithVic

Expert blogs

Blogs by vaping experts and academics

Clive Bates: The counterfactual
Insightful analysis by the world's leading campaigner on tobacco harm reduction and former head of Action on Smoking and Health UK.
https://www.clivebates.com/

Professor Michael Siegel: The Rest of the Story
Analysis and commentary by leading US academic.
http://tobaccoanalysis.blogspot.com.au/

Dr Konstantinos Farsalinos: E-cigarette Research
http://www.ecigarette-research.org
Scientific blog by one of the world's leading e-cigarette researchers.

Professor Brad Rodu: Tobacco Truth
Professor of Medicine with special expertise in tobacco harm reduction.
https://rodutobaccotruth.blogspot.com.au/

Dr Carl V Phillips: Tobacco harm reduction, anti-THR lies, and related topics
Blog by a prominent tobacco harm reduction advocate and scientist.
https://antithrlies.com/

QUOTES FROM LEADING HEALTH AND MEDICAL ORGANISATIONS

Royal Australian and New Zealand College of Psychiatrists

'The RANZCP acknowledges that e-cigarettes and vaporisers provide a less harmful way to deliver nicotine to people who smoke, thereby minimising the harm associated with smoking tobacco and reducing some of the health disparities experienced by people living with mental illness.'

Position Statement, October 2018[400]

Royal Australian College of General Practitioners

'For people who have tried to achieve smoking cessation with first-line therapy (combination of behavioural support and TGA-approved pharmacotherapy) but failed and are still motivated to quit smoking, NVPs [Nicotine Vaping Products] may be a reasonable intervention to recommend along with behavioural support.'

Supporting smoking cessation: A guide for health professionals, 2021[4]

British Medical Association

'There are clear potential benefits to their use in reducing the substantial harms associated with smoking, and a growing consensus that they are significantly less harmful than tobacco use.'

Position Paper 2017[417]

New Zealand Ministry of Health

'Expert opinion is that vaping products are much less harmful than smoking tobacco but not completely harmless. A range of toxicants have been found in vapour including some cancer-causing agents but, in general, at levels much lower than found in cigarette smoke or at levels that are unlikely to cause harm. Smokers switching to vaping products are highly likely to reduce the risks to their health and those around them. Vaping products release negligible levels of nicotine and other toxicants into ambient air with no identified health risks to bystanders.'

Position Statement on vaping 2020[244]

US National Academies of Sciences, Engineering and Medicine

'There is conclusive evidence that completely substituting e-cigarettes for combustible tobacco cigarettes reduces users' exposure to numerous toxicants and carcinogens present in combustible tobacco cigarettes.'

'There is substantial evidence that completely switching from regular use of combustible tobacco cigarettes to e-cigarettes results in reduced short-term adverse health outcomes in several organ systems.'

The Public Health Consequences of E-Cigarettes 2018[85]

Health Canada

'Vaping is less harmful than smoking. Completely replacing cigarette smoking with vaping will reduce your exposure to harmful chemicals. While evidence is still emerging, some evidence suggests that using e-cigarettes is linked to improved rates of success.'

Health Canada website, June 2021[88]

French National Academy of Medicine

'The e-cigarette is less dangerous than cigarettes and helps to stop and reduce tobacco consumption. 700,000 smokers have quit thanks to it.'

Press release, December 2019[418]

National Health Service, England

E-cigarettes are 'far less harmful than cigarettes and can help you quit smoking for good.'

NHS website, March 2019[45]

Public Health England

'on current evidence, there is no doubt that smokers who switch to vaping reduce the risks to their health dramatically.'

Online statement [84]

HEALTH AND MEDICAL
ORGANISATIONS SUPPORTING VAPING

Australia

- Royal Australian and New Zealand College of Psychiatrists
- Royal Australian College of General Practitioners
- Harm Reduction Australia
- Australian Tobacco Harm Reduction Association (ATHRA)

United Kingdom

- Royal College of Physicians, UK
- Public Health England
- British Lung Foundation
- British Heart Foundation
- British Medical Association
- Royal College of General Practitioners
- British Thoracic Society
- Royal College of Psychiatrists
- Cancer Research UK
- British Psychological Society
- Royal Society for Public Health
- National Institute for Health and Care Excellence

- The Royal College of Midwives
- Royal College of Nursing
- National Health Service, England
- Cochrane Tobacco Addiction Review Group
- Action on Smoking and Health UK
- UK Centre for Tobacco and Alcohol Studies
- National Centre for Smoking Cessation and Training
- Smoking in Pregnancy Challenge group
- National Health Service, Scotland
- Action on Smoking and Health Scotland
- Mental Health and Smoking Partnership
- Society for the Study of Addiction

New Zealand

- New Zealand Ministry of Health
- New Zealand Medical Association
- Heart Foundation New Zealand
- Cancer Society of New Zealand
- Action on Smoking and Health NZ
- Hapai te hauora. Maori Public Health
- Quitline NZ
- New Zealand College of Midwives
- Health Promotion Agency
- National Training Service (NTS)
- Pharmacy Guild of New Zealand
- All District Health Boards
- End Smoking New Zealand
- Parents Centre
- Vape2save

Canada

- Canadian Institute for Substance Use Research
- Health Canada
- Centre for Addiction and Mental Health
- Centre for Effective Practice

France

- French National Academy of Medicine

United States of America

- National Academies of Sciences, Engineering Medicine
- American Heart Association
- American Council on Science and Health

ACKNOWLEDGEMENTS

I am grateful to the many people who have helped in the writing of this book and for reviewing it to ensure its accuracy.

Special thanks to tobacco and harm reduction experts Dr Alex Wodak AM, Professor Wayne Hall and Louise Ross (UK) who generously gave their time to review all aspects of the book and give valuable feedback.

Specific sections were also reviewed by leading advocate Clive Bates (UK), Professor Chris Bullen (NZ), Professor Hayden McRobbie (NZ), Professor Peter Hajek (UK), toxicologist Eliana Golberstein (NZ), DIY expert Pippa Starr, Dr Jacques Le Houezec (France) and Professor Neal Benowitz (US).

I am very grateful to Australian industry experts and vape shop vendors for their advice on devices and e-liquids. Thank you Savvas Dimitriou, Mal Bodie, Andrew Cameron, Maxim Fichkin, Shea Williams-Philpott, Ben Pryor, Jimmy Jones and Rhys Callender. Katie Dillon gave valuable input and helped me access some of the images. Most industry experts are past or current vapers and they also provided expert advice on vaping generally.

Thanks also to GPs Dr Carolyn Beaumont, Dr Gillian Deakin, Dr Brad McKay, Dr Peter Holloway and Dr Joe Kosterich for their feedback from the general practice perspective; men's health specialist Dr Michael Lowy; and vaping guru Steve Rehberger from Legion Vapes. Valuable feedback from vapers Mike Sandic and Adam Metelmann was also very helpful.

My wife Sue reviewed every section, provided valuable input and put up with my long hours spent on the book when I should have been doing other things. My brother Martyn provided the great book title and other very helpful and insightful suggestions. Richard Sauerman, a vaper and branding expert came up with the idea for the cover.

Alex Wodak has been a friend and inspirational colleague in the campaign to legalise vaping in Australia. His thirty years of campaigning for drug harm reduction have provided valuable insights and I am very grateful for his support and wise counsel.

I also owe a great debt to Clive Bates from the UK who has tirelessly led the global campaign to recognise vaping as a lifesaving tool for smokers. Clive has generously provided guidance, advice and practical support to me and a wide network of tobacco harm reduction advocates over many years. Without his extraordinary vision, vaping would be in a very different place.

I must also mention the leading researchers who have provided the hard science which underpins vaping. These include Konstantinos Farsalinos, Riccardo Polosa, Peter Hajek, David Abrams, Ken Warner, Anne McNeill, John Britton, Maciej Goniewicz, Robert West, Jamie Brown, Lion Shahab, Hayden McRobbie, Neal Benowitz, Coral Gartner and Ron Borland, to name just a few. My apologies to the many others who are not mentioned.

Thank you to my publisher Linda Lycett and her team at Aurora House, Lucy, Marion and Donika, who have provided good advice and patiently accepted my endless corrections. It is often not easy working with an impatient perfectionist like me!

My grateful thanks to all the vapers who agreed to tell their stories, often revealing personal information in the cause of helping other smokers quit.

Last but not least, thank you Professor Robyn Richmond. Robyn sparked my interest in smoking cessation in the 1980s and has been an inspiring teacher, mentor, supporter and example for me over many years. I have been addicted to smoking cessation ever since.

REFERENCES

1. Australian Instiue of Health and Welfare. Burden of tobacco use in Australia: Australian Burden of Disease Study 2015. Australian Burden of Disease series no. 21. Cat. no. BOD 20. Canberra: AIHW. 2019. Available from: https://www.aihw.gov.au/reports/burden-of-disease/burden-of-tobacco-use-in-australia/contents/table-of-contents.

2. Banks E et al. Tobacco smoking and all-cause mortality in a large Australian cohort study: findings from a mature epidemic with current low smoking prevalence. *BMC Med*. 2015

3. Mendelsohn CP. Electronic cigarettes: what can we learn from the UK experience? *Med J Aust*. 2016

4. Royal Australian College of General Practitioners. Supporting smoking cessation: A guide for health professionals 2021. Available from: https://www.racgp.org.au/supporting-smoking-cessation.

5. Australian Instiue of Health and Welfare. National Drug Strategy Household Survey 2019. Drug Statistics series no. 32. PHE 270. Canberra AIHW. 2020. Available from: https://www.aihw.gov.au/reports/illicit-use-of-drugs/national-drug-strategy-household-survey-2019/contents/summary.

6. West R et al. Smoking Toolkit Study. Smoking in England 2021. Available from: https://smokinginengland.info/graphs/e-cigarettes-latest-trends.

7. Caraballo RS et al. Quit Methods Used by US Adult Cigarette Smokers, 2014-2016. *Prev Chronic Dis*. 2017

8. European Commission. Special Eurobarometer 458. Attitudes of Europeans towards tobacco and electronic cigarettes 2017. Available from: https://data.europa.eu/euodp/en/data/dataset/S2146_87_1_458_ENG.

9. Hartmann-Boyce J et al. Electronic cigarettes for smoking cessation. *Cochrane Database Syst Rev*. 2021

10. Notley C et al. The unique contribution of e-cigarettes for tobacco harm reduction in supporting smoking relapse prevention. *Harm Reduct J*. 2018

11. U.S. Department of Health and Human Services. How Tobacco Smoke Causes Disease: The Biology and Behavioural Basis for Smoking of Attributable Disease. A Report of the Surgeon General. Atlanta, GA: U.S. Department of Health and Human Services, Centers for Disease Control and Prevention, National Center for Chronic Disease Prevention and Health Promotion, Office on Smoking and Health. 2010

12. Royal College of Physicians. Nicotine without smoke: Tobacco harm reduction. London: RCP 2016 Available from: https://www.rcplondon.ac.uk/projects/outputs/ nicotine-without-smoke-tobacco-harm-reduction-0.

13. International Agency for Research on Cancer. Tobacco smoking and carcinogenic risk to humans. IARC Monograph 100E 2012. Available from: http://monographs.iarc.fr/ ENG/Monographs/vol100E/mono100E-6.pdf.

14. Benowitz NL et al. Cardiovascular effects of electronic cigarettes. *Nat Rev Cardiol.* 2017

15. US Department of Health and Human Services. The health consequences of smoking - 50 years of progress. A report of the Surgeon General. 2014. Available from: https:// www.surgeongeneral.gov/library/reports/50-years-of-progress/full-report.pdf.

16. Russell C et al. Changing patterns of first e-cigarette flavor used and current flavors used by 20,836 adult frequent e-cigarette users in the USA. *Harm Reduct J.* 2018 https://pubmed.ncbi.nlm.nih.gov/29954412https://www.ncbi.nlm.nih.gov/pmc/ articles/PMC6022703/

17. Action on Smoking and Health UK. Use of e-cigarettes among young people in Great Britain, 2020 2021. Available from: https://ash.org.uk/wp-content/uploads/2021/02/ YouthEcig2020.pdf.

18. Polosa R et al. A fresh look at tobacco harm reduction: the case for the electronic cigarette. *Harm Reduct J.* 2013

19. Shiffman S et al. Introduction to the Special Issue on JUUL Use. *Am J Health Behav.* 2021

20. Abrams DB et al. Managing nicotine without smoke to save lives now: Evidence for harm minimization. *Prev Med.* 2018

21. Nutt DJ et al. Estimating the harms of nicotine-containing products using the MCDA approach. *Eur Addict Res.* 2014

22. Abrams DB et al. Harm Minimization and Tobacco Control: Reframing Societal Views of Nicotine Use to Rapidly Save Lives. *Annu Rev Public Health.* 2018

23. Therapeutic Goods Administration. Nicotine e-cigarette access 2021. Available from: https://www.tga.gov.au/nicotine-e-cigarette-access.

24. New Zealand Ministry of Health. Vaping Facts 2020. Available from: https:// vapingfacts.health.nz.

25. Australian Institute of Health and Welfare. National Drug Strategy Household Survey (NDSHS) 2016: detailed findings. Drug Statistics series no. 31. Cat. no. PHE 214.

Canberra: AIHW 2017. Available from: https://www.aihw.gov.au/getmedia/15db8c15-7062-4cde-bfa4-3c2079f30af3/21028.pdf.aspx?inline=true.

26. Office for National Statistics. Adult smoking habits in the UK: 2019. 2020. Available from: https://www.ons.gov.uk/releases/adultsmokinghabitsintheuk2019.

27. Ministry of Health New Zealand. New Zealand Health Survey 2019. Available from: https://minhealthnz.shinyapps.io/nz-health-survey-2018-19-annual-data-explorer/.

28. Dai H et al. Prevalence of e-Cigarette Use Among Adults in the United States, 2014-2018. *JAMA*. 2019

29. Global State of Tobacco Harm Reduction. Burning Issues 2020. Available from: https://gsthr.org/resources/type/reports.

30. Numbeo. Price Rankings by Country of Cigarettes 20 Pack (Marlboro) 2020. Available from: https://www.numbeo.com/cost-of-living/country_price_rankings?displayCurrency=AUD&itemId=17.

31. Wackowski OA et al. Content Analysis of US News Stories About E-Cigarettes in 2015. *Nicotine Tob Res*. 2018 https://pubmed.ncbi.nlm.nih.gov/29065205/

32. Intergovernmental Committee on Drugs. National Tobacco Strategy 2012-2018. Publications approval number: D1013 2012. Available from: https://www.health.gov.au/resources/publications/national-tobacco-strategy-2012-2018.

33. World Health Organisation. Framework Convention on Tobacco Control (FCTC) 2003. Available from: http://apps.who.int/iris/bitstream/10665/42811/1/9241591013.pdf?ua=1.

34. Faine G. ABC interview with Jon Faine 2019. Available from: https://www.greghunt.com.au/abc-interview-with-jon-faine-3/.

35. Yong HH et al. Does the Regulatory Environment for E-Cigarettes Influence the Effectiveness of E-Cigarettes for Smoking Cessation?: Longitudinal Findings From the ITC Four Country Survey. *Nicotine Tob Res*. 2017

36. Department of Health TGA. Personal Importation Scheme 2015. Available from: https://www.tga.gov.au/personal-importation-scheme.

37. Therapeutic Goods Administration. Nicotine e-cigarettes: Questions and answers 2020. Available from: https://www.tga.gov.au/nicotine-e-cigarettes-questions-and-answers.

38. Therapeutic Goods Administration. Authorised prescribers 2021. Available from: https://www.tga.gov.au/form/authorised-prescribers.

39. Australian Tobacco Harm Reduction Association. The law 2020. Available from: www.athra.org.au/the-law/.

40. New Zealand Ministry of Health. Smokefree Environments and Regulated Products Act 1990 - Proposals for regulations 2021. Available from: https://consult.health.govt.nz/tobacco-control/vaping-regulations-consultation/.

41. Verrall A. New Zealand voices shape vaping regulations. Media release 10 August 2021. Available from: https://www.beehive.govt.nz/release/new-zealand-voices-shape-vaping-regulations.

42. New Zealand Ministry of Health. Vaping information for stop-smoking services and health workers. 2018. Available from: https://www.health.govt.nz/our-work/regulation-health-and-disability-system/regulation-vaping-and-smokeless-tobacco-products/vaping-information-specific-audiences/vaping-information-stop-smoking-services-and-health-workers.

43. Te Hiringa Hauora/Health Promotion Agency. Vape to QuitStrong 2021. Available from: https://www.hpa.org.nz/vapetoquitstrong-resources.

44. Australian Tobacco Harm Reduction Association. UK Parliament continues to strongly endorse vaping 2019. Available from: https://www.athra.org.au/blog/2019/11/02/uk-parliament-continues-to-strongly-endorse-vaping/.

45. National Health Service UK. Using e-cigarettes to stop smoking 2019. Available from: https://www.nhs.uk/live-well/quit-smoking/using-e-cigarettes-to-stop-smoking/.

46. McNeill A et al. Vaping in England: An evidence update including vaping for smoking cessation, February 2021: a report commissioned by Public Health England. London: Public Health England 2021. Available from: https://assets.publishing.service.gov.uk/government/uploads/system/uploads/attachment_data/file/962221/Vaping_in_England_evidence_update_February_2021.pdf.

47. Public Health England. Stoptober 2020. Available from: https://campaignresources.phe.gov.uk/resources/.

48. Steinberg MB et al. Nicotine Risk Misperception Among US Physicians. *J Gen Intern Med*. 2020

49. Tushingham S et al. Biomolecular archaeology reveals ancient origins of indigenous tobacco smoking in North American Plateau. *Proc Natl Acad Sci U S A*. 2018

50. Ratsch A et al. The pituri story: a review of the historical literature surrounding traditional Australian Aboriginal use of nicotine in Central Australia. *J Ethnobiol Ethnomed*. 2010

51. Benowitz NL. Clinical pharmacology of nicotine: implications for understanding, preventing, and treating tobacco addiction. *Clin Pharmacol Ther*. 2008

52. National Institute on Drug Abuse. Tolerance, Dependence, Addiction: What's the Difference? 2017. Available from: https://archives.drugabuse.gov/blog/post/tolerance-dependence-addiction-whats-difference.

53. Russell MA. Low-tar medium-nicotine cigarettes: a new approach to safer smoking. *Br Med J*. 1976

54. Royal Society for Public Health. Nicotine no more harmful to health than caffeine 2015. Available from: https://www.rsph.org.uk/about-us/news/nicotine--no-more-harmful-to-health-than-caffeine-.html.

55. McNeill A et al. Evidence review of e-cigarettes and heated tobacco products 2018. A report commissioned by Public Health England. London: Public Health England 2018. Available from: https://www.gov.uk/government/publications/e-cigarettes-and-heated-tobacco-products-evidence-review.

56. Hartmann-Boyce J et al. Nicotine replacement therapy versus control for smoking cessation. *Cochrane Database Syst Rev.* 2018

57. Benowitz NL. Pharmacology of nicotine: addiction, smoking-induced disease, and therapeutics. *Annu Rev Pharmacol Toxicol.* 2009

58. Maina G et al. Transdermal nicotine absorption handling e-cigarette refill liquids. *Regul Toxicol Pharmacol.* 2016

59. Ramstrom L et al. Patterns of Smoking and Snus Use in Sweden: Implications for Public Health. *Int J Environ Res Public Health.* 2016

60. Ramstrom L et al. Mortality attributable to tobacco among men in Sweden and other European countries: an analysis of data in a WHO report. *Tob Induc Dis.* 2014

61. Benowitz NL et al. Nicotine chemistry, metabolism, kinetics and biomarkers. *Handb Exp Pharmacol.* 2009

62. Shiffman S et al. Dependence on e-cigarettes and cigarettes in a cross-sectional study of US adults. *Addiction.* 2020

63. Hajek P et al. Dependence potential of nicotine replacement treatments: effects of product type, patient characteristics, and cost to user. *Prev Med.* 2007

64. West R et al. Health-care interventions to promote and assist tobacco cessation: a review of efficacy, effectiveness and affordability for use in national guideline development. *Addiction.* 2015

65. Mendelsohn C. Optimising nicotine replacement therapy in clinical practice. *Aust Fam Physician.* 2013

66. Barbeau AM et al. Perceived efficacy of e-cigarettes versus nicotine replacement therapy among successful e-cigarette users: a qualitative approach. *Addict Sci Clin Pract.* 2013

67. Bar-Zeev Y et al. Nicotine replacement therapy for smoking cessation during pregnancy. *Med J Aust.* 2018

68. Claire R et al. Pharmacological interventions for promoting smoking cessation during pregnancy. *Cochrane Database Syst Rev.* 2020

69. Blanc J et al. Nicotine Replacement Therapy during Pregnancy and Child Health Outcomes: A Systematic Review. *Int J Environ Res Public Health.* 2021

70. Zwar N et al. Nicotine and nicotine replacement therapy – the facts. *Australian Pharmacist.* 2006

71. Benowitz NL. Nicotine addiction. *N Engl J Med.* 2010

72. Heishman SJ et al. Meta-analysis of the acute effects of nicotine and smoking on human performance. *Psychopharmacology (Berl)*. 2010

73. Morissette SB et al. Anxiety, anxiety disorders, tobacco use, and nicotine: a critical review of interrelationships. *Psychol Bull*. 2007

74. Tian J et al. The association between quitting smoking and weight gain: a systemic review and meta-analysis of prospective cohort studies. *Obes Rev*. 2015

75. Glover M et al. Could Vaping be a New Weapon in the Battle of the Bulge? *Nicotine Tob Res*. 2016

76. Featherstone RE et al. The Role of Nicotine in Schizophrenia. *Int Rev Neurobiol*. 2015

77. Potter AS et al. Acute nicotine improves cognitive deficits in young adults with attention-deficit/hyperactivity disorder. *Pharmacol Biochem Behav*. 2008

78. Covey LS et al. Anxiety and Depressed Mood Decline Following Smoking Abstinence in Adult Smokers with Attention Deficit Hyperactivity Disorder. *J Subst Abuse Treat*. 2015

79. Alhowail A. Molecular insights into the benefits of nicotine on memory and cognition (Review). *Mol Med Rep*. 2021

80. Ma C et al. Nicotine from cigarette smoking and diet and Parkinson disease: a review. *Transl Neurodegener*. 2017

81. Lunney PC et al. Review article: Ulcerative colitis, smoking and nicotine therapy. *Aliment Pharmacol Ther*. 2012

82. Carstens E E et al. Sensory effects of nicotine and tobacco. *Nicotine & Tobacco Research*. 2021 https://doi.org/10.1093/ntr/ntab086

83. Goniewicz ML et al. Levels of selected carcinogens and toxicants in vapour from electronic cigarettes. *Tob Control*. 2014

84. McNeill A et al. E-cigarettes: an evidence update. A report commissioned by Public Health England. PHE publications gateway number: 2015260. 2015. Available at https://www.gov.uk/government/publications/e-cigarettes-an-evidence-update

85. National Academies of Sciences Engineering and Medicine. Public health consequences of e-cigarettes. Washington, DC: The National Academies Press 2018. Available from: http://nap.edu/24952.

86. Committee on Toxicity of Chemicals in Food Consumer products and the Environment (COT). Statement on the potential toxicological risks from electronic nicotine (and non-nicotine) delivery systems (E(N)NDS – e-cigarettes) 2020. Available from: https://cot.food.gov.uk/sites/default/files/2020-09/COT%20E%28N%29NDS%20statement%20 2020-04.pdf.

87. Centre for Addiction and Mental Health. Lower-Risk Nicotine Use Guidelines. Funded by Health Canada 2021. Available from: https://www.nicotinedependenceclinic.com/ en/Pages/Lower-Risk-Nicotine-Use-Guidelin%E2%80%8Bes.aspx.

88. Health Canada. Vaping and quitting smoking 2021. Available from: https://www. canada.ca/en/health-canada/services/smoking-tobacco/vaping/smokers.html.

89. Eissenberg T et al. Invalidity of an Oft-Cited Estimate of the Relative Harms of Electronic Cigarettes. *Am J Public Health*. 2020

90. Goniewicz ML et al. Comparison of Nicotine and Toxicant Exposure in Users of Electronic Cigarettes and Combustible Cigarettes. *JAMA Netw Open*. 2018

91. George J et al. Cardiovascular Effects of Switching From Tobacco Cigarettes to Electronic Cigarettes. *J Am Coll Cardiol*. 2019

92. Farsalinos K et al. Effect of continuous smoking reduction and abstinence on blood pressure and heart rate in smokers switching to electronic cigarettes. *Intern Emerg Med*. 2016

93. Polosa R et al. Persisting long term benefits of smoking abstinence and reduction in asthmatic smokers who have switched to electronic cigarettes. *Discov Med*. 2016

94. Polosa R et al. COPD smokers who switched to e-cigarettes: health outcomes at 5-year follow up. *Ther Adv Chronic Dis*. 2020

95. Kosmider L et al. Carbonyl compounds in electronic cigarette vapors: effects of nicotine solvent and battery output voltage. *Nicotine Tob Res*. 2014

96. Stephens WE. Comparing the cancer potencies of emissions from vapourised nicotine products including e-cigarettes with those of tobacco smoke. *Tob Control*. 2017 DOI: 10.1136/tobaccocontrol-2017-053808 [Epub ahead of print]

97. McNeill A et al. Underpinning evidence for the estimate that e-cigarette use is around 95% safer than smoking: authors' note. PHE publications gateway: 2015260 2015. Available from: https://www.gov.uk/government/publications/e-cigarettes-an-evidence-update.

98. Shahab L et al. Nicotine, Carcinogen, and Toxin Exposure in Long-Term E-Cigarette and Nicotine Replacement Therapy Users: A Cross-sectional Study. *Ann Intern Med*. 2017

99. Thorne D et al. The mutagenic assessment of an electronic-cigarette and reference cigarette smoke using the Ames assay in strains TA98 and TA100. *Mutat Res Genet Toxicol Environ Mutagen*. 2016

100. Scungio M et al. Measurements of electronic cigarette-generated particles for the evaluation of lung cancer risk of active and passive users. *Journal of Aerosol Science*. 2018

101. Benowitz NL et al. Cardiovascular toxicity of nicotine: Implications for electronic cigarette use. *Trends Cardiovasc Med*. 2016

102. Hubbard R et al. Use of nicotine replacement therapy and the risk of acute myocardial infarction, stroke, and death. *Tob Control*. 2005

103. Rostron BL et al. Smokeless tobacco use and circulatory disease risk: a systematic review and meta-analysis. *Open Heart*. 2018

104. Münzel T et al. Effects of tobacco cigarettes, e-cigarettes, and waterpipe smoking on endothelial function and clinical outcomes. *Eur Heart J*. 2020

105. Middlekauff HR. Cardiovascular impact of electronic-cigarette use. *Trends Cardiovasc Med*. 2020

106. Bhatta DN et al. Electronic Cigarette Use and Myocardial Infarction Among Adults in the US Population Assessment of Tobacco and Health. *J Am Heart Assoc*. 2019

107. Wills TA et al. E-cigarette use and respiratory disorders: an integrative review of converging evidence from epidemiological and laboratory studies. *Eur Respir J*. 2021

108. Hajek P et al. A randomised trial of e-cigarettes versus nicotine replacement therapy. *N Engl J Med*. 2019

109. Farsalinos KE et al. Characteristics, perceived side effects and benefits of electronic cigarette use: a worldwide survey of more than 19,000 consumers. *Int J Environ Res Public Health*. 2014

110. Polosa R et al. Effect of smoking abstinence and reduction in asthmatic smokers switching to electronic cigarettes: evidence for harm reversal. *Int J Environ Res Public Health*. 2014

111. Miler J et al. Changes in the Frequency of Airway Infections in Smokers Who Switched To Vaping: Results of an Online Survey. *Journal of Addiction Research & Therapy*. 2016

112. Jose T et al. Electronic Cigarette Use Is Not Associated with COVID-19 Diagnosis. *J Prim Care Community Health*. 2021

113. Shanks N et al. Are animal models predictive for humans? *Philos Ethics Humanit Med*. 2009

114. Bhatta DN et al. Association of E-Cigarette Use With Respiratory Disease Among Adults: A Longitudinal Analysis. *Am J Prev Med*. 2020

115. Kenkel D et al. E-cigarettes and respiratory disease: a replication, extension and future directions. Working Paper 27507 2020. Available from: https://www.nber.org/system/files/working_papers/w27507/w27507.pdf.

116. Cancer Research UK. Does vaping cause popcorn lung? 2018. Available from: https://www.cancerresearchuk.org/about-cancer/causes-of-cancer/does-vaping-cause-popcorn-lung.

117. Siegel M. New Study Finds that Average Diacetyl Exposure from Vaping is 750 Times Lower than from Smoking 2015. Available from: http://tobaccoanalysis.blogspot.com/2015/12/new-study-finds-that-average-diacetyl.html.

118. Australian Government Department of Health. Therapeutic Goods (Standard for Nicotine Vaping Products) (TGO110) Order 2021 (TGO110) 2021. Available from: https://www.legislation.gov.au/Details/F2021L00595.

119. Blount BC et al. Vitamin E Acetate in Bronchoalveolar-Lavage Fluid Associated with EVALI. *N Engl J Med*. 2019

120. Centers for Disease Control and Prevention. Outbreak of Lung Injury Associated with E-cigarette Use, or Vaping 2020. Available from: https://www.cdc.gov/tobacco/basic_information/e-cigarettes/severe-lung-disease.html.

121. Hall W et al. Lessons from the public health responses to the US outbreak of vaping-related lung injury. *Addiction*. 2020

122. St Helen G et al. Nicotine delivery, retention and pharmacokinetics from various electronic cigarettes. *Addiction*. 2016

123. Martuzevicius D et al. Characterisation of the Spatial and Temporal Dispersion Differences between Exhaled e-cigarette mist and Cigarette Smoke. *Nicotine Tob Res*. 2018

124. Avino P et al. Second-hand aerosol from tobacco and electronic cigarettes: Evaluation of the smoker emission rates and doses and lung cancer risk of passive smokers and vapers. *Sci Total Environ*. 2018

125. Levy DT et al. Examining the relationship of vaping to smoking initiation among US youth and young adults: a reality check. *Tob Control*. 2019

126. The Royal College of Midwives. Position Statement. Support to Quit Smoking in Pregnancy 2019. Available from: https://www.rcm.org.uk/media/3394/support-to-quit-smoking-in-pregnancy.pdf.

127. England LJ et al. Adverse pregnancy outcomes in snuff users. *Am J Obstet Gynecol*. 2003

128. Nardone N et al. JUUL electronic cigarettes: Nicotine exposure and the user experience. *Drug Alcohol Depend*. 2019

129. Smith TT et al. Effects of Monoamine Oxidase Inhibition on the Reinforcing Properties of Low-Dose Nicotine. *Neuropsychopharmacology*. 2016

130. West R et al. Epidemic of youth nicotine addiction? What does the National Youth Tobacco Survey reveal about high school ecigarette use in the USA? 2019. Available from: https://www.qeios.com/read/article/391.

131. Wylie C et al. Exposures to e-cigarettes and their refills: calls to Australian Poisons Information Centres, 2009–2016. *Medical Journal of Australia*. 2019

132. Australian Tobacco Harm Reduction Association. Health Minister misinformed about nicotine poisoning 2020. Available from: https://www.athra.org.au/blog/2020/09/05/health-minister-misinformed-about-nicotine-poisoning/.

133. Australian Tobacco Harm Reduction Association. Tragic death of child highlights urgent need for liquid nicotine regulation 2020. Available from: https://www.athra.org.au/blog/media_releases/tragic-death-of-child-highlights-urgent-need-for-liquid-nicotine-regulation/.

134. Gummin DD et al. 2018 Annual Report of the American Association of Poison Control Centers' National Poison Data System (NPDS): 36th Annual Report. *Clin Toxicol (Phila)*. 2019

135. UK Government. e-cigarettes and refill containers (e-liquids): report suspected side effects and safety concerns 2017. Available from: https://www.gov.uk/drug-safety-update/e-cigarettes-and-refill-containers-e-liquids-report-suspected-side-effects-and-safety-concerns.

136. McFaull SR et al. Injuries and poisonings associated with e-cigarettes and vaping substances, electronic Canadian Hospitals Injury Reporting and Prevention Program, 2011-2019. *Health Promot Chronic Dis Prev Can*. 2020

137. Scarpino M et al. Brain death following ingestion of E-cigarette liquid nicotine refill solution. *Brain Behav*. 2020

138. Cairns R et al. Paracetamol poisoning-related hospital admissions and deaths in Australia, 2004-2017. *Med J Aust*. 2019

139. Hua M et al. Potential health effects of electronic cigarettes: A systematic review of case reports. *Prev Med Rep*. 2016

140. Vyncke T et al. Injuries associated with electronic nicotine delivery systems: a systematic review. *J Trauma Acute Care Surg*. 2020

141. Mankowski PJ et al. Cellular phone collateral damage: A review of burns associated with lithium battery powered mobile devices. *Burns*. 2016

142. Royal College of Physicians TAG. Smoking and health 2021: A coming of age for tobacco control? 2021. Available from: https://www.rcplondon.ac.uk/projects/outputs/smoking-and-health-2021-coming-age-tobacco-control.

143. Lawlor DA et al. Triangulation in aetiological epidemiology. *Int J Epidemiol*. 2016

144. Walker N et al. Nicotine patches used in combination with e-cigarettes (with and without nicotine) for smoking cessation: a pragmatic, randomised trial. *Lancet Respir Med*. 2019

145. Hartmann-Boyce J et al. Electronic cigarettes for smoking cessation. *Cochrane Database Syst Rev*. 2021

146. Grabovac I et al. Effectiveness of Electronic Cigarettes in Smoking Cessation: a Systematic Review and Meta-Analysis. *Nicotine Tob Res*. 2020

147. The Joanna Briggs Institute. E–cigarettes for smoking cessation guideline update: technical report of evidence review and summary of findings 2019. Available from: https://www.racgp.org.au/getmedia/2e90f512-a8a8-4c89-b226-56ada993c7f1/ECigarettes-for-Smoking-Cessation-Technical-Report.pdf.aspx.

148. Chan GCK et al. A systematic review of randomized controlled trials and network meta-analysis of e-cigarettes for smoking cessation. *Addict Behav*. 2021

149. Banks E et al. Systematic review and meta-analysis of evidence on the efficacy of e-cigarette use for sustained smoking and nicotine cessation. Medrxiv. 2020. Available from: https://www.medrxiv.org/content/10.1101/2020.11.02.20224212v1.

150. Pound CM et al. Smoking cessation in individuals who use vaping as compared with traditional nicotine replacement therapies: a systematic review and meta-analysis. *BMJ Open*. 2021

151. Lee SH et al. Effect of Electronic Cigarettes on Smoking Reduction and Cessation in Korean Male Smokers: A Randomized Controlled Study. *J Am Board Fam Med*. 2019

152. Wang RJ et al. E-Cigarette Use and Adult Cigarette Smoking Cessation: A Meta-Analysis. *Am J Public Health*. 2021

153. Berry KM et al. E-cigarette initiation and associated changes in smoking cessation and reduction: the Population Assessment of Tobacco and Health Study, 2013-2015. *Tob Control*. 2018

154. Hitchman SC et al. Associations Between E-Cigarette Type, Frequency of Use, and Quitting Smoking: Findings From a Longitudinal Online Panel Survey in Great Britain. *Nicotine Tob Res*. 2015

155. Phillips CV. Science Lesson: Clinical Trials Are A Terrible Way To Assess Vaping 2017. Available from: http://dailyvaper.com/2017/12/11/science-lesson-clinical-trials-are-a-terrible-way-to-assess-vaping/.

156. Thompson A. The Accidental Quitter & Why They Are Important 2019. Available from: https://thethr.blog/accidental-quitter/.

157. Foulds J et al. Effect of Electronic Nicotine Delivery Systems on Cigarette Abstinence in Smokers with no Plans to Quit: Exploratory Analysis of a Randomized Placebo-Controlled Trial. *MedRxiv*. 2021 https://www.medrxiv.org/content/10.1101/2021.06.22.21259359v1.full.pdf+html

158. Glasser AM et al. Overview of Electronic Nicotine Delivery Systems: A Systematic Review. *Am J Prev Med*. 2017

159. Villanti AC et al. How do we determine the impact of e-cigarettes on cigarette smoking cessation or reduction? Review and recommendations for answering the research question with scientific rigor. *Addiction*. 2017

160. Zhu SH et al. E-cigarette use and associated changes in population smoking cessation: evidence from US current population surveys. *BMJ*. 2017

161. Johnson L et al. E-cigarette Usage Is Associated With Increased Past-12-Month Quit Attempts and Successful Smoking Cessation in Two US Population-Based Surveys. *Nicotine Tob Res*. 2018

162. Beard E et al. Association of prevalence of electronic cigarette use with smoking cessation and cigarette consumption in England: a time series analysis between 2006 and 2017. *Addiction*. 2019

163. Giovenco DP et al. Prevalence of population smoking cessation by electronic cigarette use status in a national sample of recent smokers. *Addict Behav.* 2017

164. World Vapers' Alliance. From Smoking to Vaping - Lives Saved 2021. Available from: https://worldvapersalliance.com/from-smoking-to-vaping/.

165. Friedman AS. How does electronic cigarette access affect adolescent smoking? *J Health Econ.* 2015

166. Pesko MF et al. The influence of electronic cigarette age purchasing restrictions on adolescent tobacco and marijuana use. *Prev Med.* 2016

167. Levy DT et al. US Nicotine Vaping Product SimSmoke Simulation Model: The Effect of Vaping and Tobacco Control Policies on Smoking Prevalence and Smoking-Attributable Deaths. *Int J Environ Res Public Health.* 2021

168. Levy DT et al. England SimSmoke: The Impact of Nicotine Vaping on Smoking Prevalence and Smoking-Attributable Deaths in England. *Addiction.* 2020

169. Livingstone-Banks J et al. Relapse prevention interventions for smoking cessation. *Cochrane Database Syst Rev.* 2019

170. Notley C et al. Vaping as an alternative to smoking relapse following brief lapse. *Drug Alcohol Rev.* 2019

171. Morphett K et al. Barriers and facilitators to switching from smoking to vaping: Advice from vapers. *Drug Alcohol Rev.* 2019

172. Russell C et al. Advice From Former-Smoking E-Cigarette Users to Current Smokers on How to Use E-Cigarettes as Part of an Attempt to Quit Smoking. *Nicotine Tob Res.* 2018

173. Ward E et al. A Qualitative Exploration of the Role of Vape Shop Environments in Supporting Smoking Abstinence. *Int J Environ Res Public Health.* 2018

174. Polosa R et al. Quit and smoking reduction rates in vape shop consumers: a prospective 12-month survey. *Int J Environ Res Public Health.* 2015

175. Wagener TL et al. Examining the Smoking and Vaping Behaviors and Preferences of Vape Shop Customers. *Tobacco Prevention & Cessation.* 2016

176. Gravely S et al. Discussions between health professionals and smokers about nicotine vaping products: results from the 2016 ITC Four Country Smoking and Vaping Survey. *Addiction.* 2019

177. Erku DA et al. Beliefs and Self-reported Practices of Health Care Professionals Regarding Electronic Nicotine Delivery Systems: A Mixed-Methods Systematic Review and Synthesis. *Nicotine Tob Res.* 2020

178. Cancer Research UK. Headlines saying 'vaping might cause cancer' are wildly misleading 2018. Available from: http://scienceblog.cancerresearchuk.org/2018/01/30/headlines-saying-vaping-might-cause-cancer-are-wildly-misleading/.

179. Cancer Research UK. 6 tips to spot cancer 'fake news' 2018. Available from: https://medicalxpress.com/news/2018-05-cancer-fake-news.html.

180. Kosmider L et al. Compensatory puffing with lower nicotine concentration e-liquids increases carbonyl exposure in e-cigarette aerosols *Nicotine Tob Res*. 2017

181. Prochaska JJ et al. Nicotine delivery and cigarette equivalents from vaping a JUULpod. *Tob Control*. 2021

182. Goldenson NI et al. Switching away from Cigarettes across 12 Months among Adult Smokers Purchasing the JUUL System. *Am J Health Behav*. 2021

183. Heatherton TF et al. Measuring the heaviness of smoking: using self-reported time to the first cigarette of the day and number of cigarettes smoked per day. *Br J Addict*. 1989

184. Hajek P et al. Nicotine delivery and users' reactions to Juul compared with cigarettes and other e-cigarette products. *Addiction*. 2020

185. Bertrand P et al. Physical and chemical assessment of 1,3 Propanediol as a potential substitute of propylene glycol in refill liquid for electronic cigarettes. *Sci Rep*. 2018

186. Benowitz NL et al. Clinical Pharmacology of Electronic Nicotine Delivery Systems (ENDS): Implications for Benefits and Risks in the Promotion of the Combusted Tobacco Endgame. *J Clin Pharmacol*. 2021

187. Glasser A et al. Patterns of e-cigarette use and subsequent cigarette smoking cessation over two years (2013/2014 to 2015/2016) in the Population Assessment of Tobacco and Health (PATH) Study. *Nicotine Tob Res*. 2020

188. Landry RL et al. The role of flavors in vaping initiation and satisfaction among U.S. adults. *Addict Behav*. 2019

189. Gendall P et al. Role of flavours in vaping uptake and cessation among New Zealand smokers and non-smokers: a cross-sectional study. *Tob Control*. 2020

190. Kreiss K et al. Clinical bronchiolitis obliterans in workers at a microwave-popcorn plant. *N Engl J Med*. 2002

191. Behar RZ et al. Distribution, quantification and toxicity of cinnamaldehyde in electronic cigarette refill fluids and aerosols. *Tob Control*. 2016

192. Kosmider L et al. Cherry-flavoured electronic cigarettes expose users to the inhalation irritant, benzaldehyde. *Thorax*. 2016

193. Scientific Committee on Health Environmental and Emerging Risks (SCHEER). Opinion on electronic cigarettes 2021. Available from: https://ec.europa.eu/health/sites/default/files/scientific_committees/scheer/docs/scheer_o_017.pdf.

194. NSW Health. RETAILER FACTSHEET. Ban on display of tobacco, smoking and e-cigarette products in retail outlets 2017. Available from: https://www.health.nsw.gov.au/tobacco/Factsheets/retailers-ban-on-display.pdf.

195. Roberts C. The End Of Mail-Order JUUL. Forbes.com 2021. Available from: https://www.forbes.com/sites/chrisroberts/2021/03/22/the-end-of-mail-order-juul-how-donald-trump-and-kamala-harris-kneecapped-vaping/?sh=12a1d1377180.

196. Therapeutic Goods Administration. Nicotine e-cigarettes: Information for prescribers 2021. Available from: https://www.tga.gov.au/nicotine-e-cigarettes-information-prescribers.

197. Australian Government. Customs Act 1901 2020. Available from: https://www.legislation.gov.au/Details/C2021C00197.

198. Therapeutic Goods Administration. Traveller's exemption 2020. Available from: https://www.tga.gov.au/entering-australia.

199. Kimber CF et al. Changes in puffing topography and subjective effects over a 2-week period in e-cigarette naïve smokers: Effects of device type and nicotine concentrations. *Addict Behav.* 2021

200. Farsalinos KE et al. Nicotine absorption from electronic cigarette use: comparison between experienced consumers (vapers) and naive users (smokers). *Sci Rep.* 2015

201. St Helen G et al. Nicotine Delivery and Vaping Behavior During ad Libitum E-cigarette Access. *Tob Regul Sci.* 2016

202. Hajek P et al. Nicotine intake from electronic cigarettes on initial use and after 4 weeks of regular use. *Nicotine Tob Res.* 2015

203. Briganti M et al. Bibliometric Analysis of Electronic Cigarette Publications: 2003⁻2018. *Int J Environ Res Public Health.* 2019

204. Wodak A. Hysteria about drugs and harm minimisation. It's always the same old story. 2016. Available from: https://www.theguardian.com/commentisfree/2016/aug/11/hysteria-about-drugs-and-harm-minimisation-its-always-the-same-old-story.

205. Balfour DJK et al. Balancing Consideration of the Risks and Benefits of E-Cigarettes. *Am J Public Health.* 2021

206. Guerin N et al. ASSAD 2017 Statistics & Trends: Australian Secondary Students' Use of Tobacco, Alcohol, Over-the-counter Drugs, and Illicit Substances. Cancer Council Victoria. 2018. Available from: https://www.health.gov.au/resources/publications/secondary-school-students-use-of-tobacco-alcohol-and-other-drugs-in-2017.

207. ASH New Zealand. ASH Year 10 Snapshot 2018. Available from: https://www.ash.org.nz/ash_year_10.

208. Bauld L et al. E-Cigarette Uptake Amongst UK Youth: Experimentation, but Little or No Regular Use in Nonsmokers. *Nicotine Tob Res.* 2016

209. Glasser AM et al. Youth Vaping and Tobacco Use in Context in the United States: Results from the 2018 National Youth Tobacco Survey. *Nicotine Tob Res.* 2020

210. de Lacy E et al. Cross-sectional study examining the prevalence, correlates and sequencing of electronic cigarette and tobacco use among 11-16-year olds in schools in Wales. *BMJ Open*. 2017

211. Jarvis M et al. Epidemic of youth nicotine addiction? What does the National Youth Tobacco Survey 2017-2019 reveal about high school e-cigarette use in the USA? Qeios 2020. Available from: https://www.qeios.com/read/745076.5/pdf.

212. Mendelsohn CP et al. Does the gateway theory justify a ban on nicotine vaping in Australia? *Int J Drug Policy*. 2020

213. Soneji S et al. Association Between Initial Use of e-Cigarettes and Subsequent Cigarette Smoking Among Adolescents and Young Adults: A Systematic Review and Meta-analysis. *JAMA Pediatr*. 2017

214. Vanyukov MM et al. Common liability to addiction and "gateway hypothesis": theoretical, empirical and evolutionary perspective. *Drug Alcohol Depend*. 2012

215. Rigsby DC et al. Electronic Vapor Product Usage and Substance Use Risk Behaviors Among U.S. High School Students. *J Child Adolesc Psychopharmacol*. 2019

216. Khouja JN et al. Association of genetic liability to smoking initiation with e-cigarette use in young adults: A cohort study. *PLoS Med*. 2021

217. Hall W et al. The "gateway" effect of e-cigarettes may be explained by a genetic liability to risk-taking. *PLoS Med*. 2021

218. New Zealand Government. New vaping to quit smoking website launches 2019. Available from: https://www.beehive.govt.nz/release/new-vaping-quit-smoking-website-launches.

219. Kozlowski LT et al. Adolescents and e-cigarettes: Objects of concern may appear larger than they are. *Drug Alcohol Depend*. 2017 https://pubmed.ncbi.nlm.nih.gov/29350617

220. Chan GCK et al. Gateway or common liability? A systematic review and meta-analysis of studies of adolescent e-cigarette use and future smoking initiation. *Addiction*. 2020

221. Kozlowski LT et al. Obsolete tobacco control themes can be hazardous to public health: the need for updating views on absolute product risks and harm reduction. *BMC Public Health*. 2016

222. Selya AS et al. Trends in electronic cigarette use and conventional smoking: quantifying a possible 'diversion' effect among US adolescents. *Addiction*. 2021

223. Foxon F et al. Electronic cigarettes, nicotine use trends and use initiation ages among US adolescents from 1999 to 2018. *Addiction*. 2020

224. Friedman AS et al. Associations of Flavored e-Cigarette Uptake With Subsequent Smoking Initiation and Cessation. *JAMA Netw Open*. 2020

225. Wang TW et al. Tobacco Product Use and Associated Factors Among Middle and High School Students - United States, 2019. *Morbidity and mortality weekly report Surveillance summaries (Washington, DC : 2002)*. 2019 https://pubmed.ncbi.nlm.nih. gov/31805035

226. Sun T et al. Has increased youth e-cigarette use in the USA, between 2014 and 2020, changed conventional smoking behaviors, future intentions to smoke and perceived smoking harms? *Addict Behav*. 2021

227. Walker N et al. Use of e-cigarettes and smoked tobacco in youth aged 14-15 years in New Zealand: findings from repeated cross-sectional studies (2014-19). *Lancet Public Health*. 2020

228. Sokol NA et al. High school seniors who used e-cigarettes may have otherwise been cigarette smokers: Evidence from Monitoring the Future (United States, 2009-2018). *Nicotine Tob Res*. 2021

229. Shahab L et al. Association of initial e-cigarette and other tobacco product use with subsequent cigarette smoking in adolescents: a cross-sectional, matched control study. *Tob Control*. 2020

230. Action on Smoking and Health UK. Use of e-cigarettes among young people in Great Britain 2019. Available from: https://www.drugsandalcohol.ie/30694/1/ASH-Factsheet-Youth-E-cigarette-Use-2019.pdf.

231. Miech R et al. What are kids vaping? Results from a national survey of US adolescents. *Tob Control*. 2017

232. Tokle R et al. Adolescents' use of nicotine-free and nicotine e-cigarettes: A longitudinal study of vaping transitions and vaper characteristics. *Nicotine Tob Res*. 2021

233. Jackson SE et al. Dependence on nicotine in US high school students in the context of changing patterns of tobacco product use. *Addiction*. 2021

234. Yuan M et al. Nicotine and the adolescent brain. *J Physiol*. 2015

235. US Department of Health and Human Services. E-Cigarette Use Among Youth and Young Adults. A Report of the Surgeon General, Atlanta, GA: U.S. Department of Health and Human Services, Centers for Disease Control and Prevention, National Center for Chronic Disease Prevention and Health Promotion, Office on Smoking and Health, 2016. https://e-cigarettes.surgeongeneral.gov/documents/2016_SGR_Full_Report_non-508.pdf.

236. Jha P et al. 21st-century hazards of smoking and benefits of cessation in the United States. *N Engl J Med*. 2013

237. Wang TW et al. Tobacco Product Use and Associated Factors Among Middle and High School Students - United States, 2019: Centers for Disease Control and Prevention; 2019. 1-22. Available from: https://www.ncbi.nlm.nih.gov/pmc/articles/PMC6903396/.

238. Park-Lee E et al. Notes from the Field: E-cigarette use among middle and high school students. National Youth Tobacco Survey US. MMWR Morb Mortal Wkly Rep 2021 2021. Available from: http://dx.doi.org/10.15585/mmwr.mm7039a4.

239. National Drug and Alcohol Research Centre - University of New South Wales. Alcohol and Young People 2016. Available from: https://ndarc.med.unsw.edu.au/sites/default/files/ndarc/resources/NDA073%20Fact%20Sheet%20Alcohol%20and%20Young%20People_0.pdf.

240. Kozlowski LT. Policy Makers and Consumers Should Prioritize Human Rights to Being Smoke-Free Over Either Tobacco- or Nicotine-Free: Accurate Terms and Relevant Evidence. *Nicotine Tob Res*. 2020

241. Baicker K et al. Evidence-Based Health Policy. *N Engl J Med*. 2017

242. Erku DA et al. Policy Debates Regarding Nicotine Vaping Products in Australia: A Qualitative Analysis of Submissions to a Government Inquiry from Health and Medical Organisations. *Int J Environ Res Public Health*. 2019

243. House of Representatives Standing Committee on Health Aged Care and Sport. Use and marketing of electronic cigarettes and personal vaporisers in Australia. Hansard 5 October 2017 2017. Available from: http://parlinfo.aph.gov.au

244. New Zealand Ministry of Health. Position Statement on Vaping 2020. Available from: https://bit.ly/2R5OW8K.

245. Saebo G et al. Assessing notions of denormalization and renormalization of smoking in light of e-cigarette regulation. *Int J Drug Policy*. 2017

246. Action on Smoking and Health UK. Use of electronic cigarettes (vapourisers) among adults in Great Britain. 2018. Available at: http://ash.org.uk/category/information-and-resources/fact-sheets/

247. European Commission. Communication on the precautionary principle. Brussels, 2.2.2000 (COM(2000) final. 2000. Available at: http://eur-lex.europa.eu/legal-content/EN/TXT/PDF/?uri=CELEX:52000DC0001&from=EN

248. Morphett K et al. The misuse of the precautionary principle in justifying Australia's ban on the sale of nicotine vaping products. *Nicotine Tob Res*. 2020

249. Mendez D et al. A magic bullet? The potential impact of e-cigarettes on the toll of cigarette smoking. *Nicotine Tob Res*. 2020

250. Petrovic-van der Deen FS et al. Potential Country-level Health and Cost Impacts of Legalizing Domestic Sale of Vaporized Nicotine Products. *Epidemiology*. 2019

251. Levy DT et al. Potential deaths averted in USA by replacing cigarettes with e-cigarettes. *Tob Control*. 2017 DOI: 10.1136/tobaccocontrol-2017-053759

252. Kotz D et al. The Use of Tobacco, E-Cigarettes, and Methods to Quit Smoking in Germany. *Dtsch Arztebl Int*. 2018

253. Kyzer L. Vaping Linked to Decrease in Cigarette Smoking. 2018 http://icelandreview.com/news/2018/05/03/vaping-linked-decrease-cigarette-smoking

254. Farsalinos KE et al. Electronic cigarette use in Greece: an analysis of a representative population sample in Attica prefecture. *Harm Reduct J*. 2018

255. Oakly A et al. Dual use of electronic cigarettes and tobacco in New Zealand from a nationally representative sample. *Aust N Z J Public Health*. 2019

256. Farsalinos KE et al. Electronic cigarette use in the European Union: analysis of a representative sample of 27 460 Europeans from 28 countries. *Addiction*. 2016

257. Selya AS et al. Dual Use of Cigarettes and JUUL: Trajectory and Cigarette Consumption. *Am J Health Behav*. 2021

258. Martinez U et al. Targeted smoking cessation for dual users of combustible and electronic cigarettes: a randomised controlled trial. *Lancet Public Health*. 2021

259. Brown J et al. Prevalence and characteristics of e-cigarette users in Great Britain: Findings from a general population survey of smokers. *Addict Behav*. 2014

260. Liu G et al. A comparison of nicotine dependence among exclusive E-cigarette and cigarette users in the PATH study. *Prev Med*. 2017

261. Piper ME et al. Changes in Use Patterns Over 1 Year Among Smokers and Dual Users of Combustible and Electronic Cigarettes. *Nicotine Tob Res*. 2020

262. Action on Smoking and Health UK. Use of e-cigarettes (vapes) among adults in Great Britain 2021. Available from: https://ash.org.uk/wp-content/uploads/2021/06/Use-of-e-cigarettes-vapes-among-adults-in-Great-Britain-2021.pdf.

263. Owusu D et al. Patterns and trends of dual use of e-cigarettes and cigarettes among U.S. adults, 2015-2018. *Prev Med Rep*. 2019

264. Arnold MJ et al. Harm reduction associated with dual use of cigarettes and e-cigarettes in Black and Latino smokers: Secondary analyses from a randomized controlled e-cigarette switching trial. *Nicotine Tob Res*. 2021

265. McRobbie H et al. Effects of Switching to Electronic Cigarettes with and without Concurrent Smoking on Exposure to Nicotine, Carbon Monoxide, and Acrolein. *Cancer Prev Res (Phila)*. 2015

266. Borland R et al. A new classification system for describing concurrent use of nicotine vaping products alongside cigarettes (so-called 'dual use'): findings from the ITC-4 Country Smoking and Vaping wave 1 Survey. *Addiction*. 2019

267. Kotz D et al. 'Real-world' effectiveness of smoking cessation treatments: a population study. *Addiction*. 2014

268. Imperial Brands. Share price 2021. Available from: https://www.imperialbrandsplc.com/investors/share-price/lse/share-chart.html.

269. Philip Morris International. 2021 Second-Quarter Results 2021. Available from: https://www.pmi.com/investor-relations/overview/event-details?EventId= 23086.

270. Action on Smoking and Health UK. Use of e-cigarettes (vapes) among adults in Great Britain 2020. Available from: https://www.drugsandalcohol.ie/33211/1/Use-of-e-cigarettes-vapes-among-adults-in-Great-Britain-2020.pdf.

271. Malt L et al. Perception of the relative harm of electronic cigarettes compared to cigarettes amongst US adults from 2013 to 2016: analysis of the Population Assessment of Tobacco and Health (PATH) study data. *Harm Reduct J.* 2020

272. Erku DA et al. Framing and scientific uncertainty in nicotine vaping product regulation: An examination of competing narratives among health and medical organisations in the UK, Australia and New Zealand. *Int J Drug Policy.* 2020

273. Kahneman D. Thinking, Fast and Slow: Penguin UK; 2012.

274. Paek H. Risk Perceptions and Risk Characteristics. Oxford Research Encyclopedias 2017. Available from: https://doi.org/10.1093/acrefore/9780190228613.013.283.

275. Ropeik D. The perception gap: An explanation for why people maintain irrational fears. 2011 https://blogs.scientificamerican.com/guest-blog/the-perception-gap-an-explanation-for-why-people-maintain-irrational-fears/

276. Bates C. The critic's guide to bad vaping science 2016. Available from: https://www.clivebates.com/the-critics-guide-to-bad-vaping-science/.

277. Haidt J. The Righteous Mind: Why Good People are Divided by Politics and Religion: Penguin Press; 2013.

278. Kozlowski LT. Minors, Moral Psychology, and the Harm Reduction Debate: The Case of Tobacco and Nicotine. *J Health Polit Policy Law.* 2017

279. Noor I. Confirmation Bias 2020. Available from: https://www.simplypsychology.org/confirmation-bias.html.

280. Swire-Thompson B et al. Searching for the Backfire Effect: Measurement and Design Considerations. *J Appl Res Mem Cogn.* 2020

281. Lord CG et al. Biased Assimilation and attitude polarization: The effects of prior theories on subsequently considered evidence. *Journal of Personality and Social Psychology.* 1979

282. Munafò MR et al. E-cigarette research needs to adopt open science practices to improve quality. *Addiction.* 2020

283. Royal College of Physicians. Harm reduction in nicotine addiction: helping people who can't quit. A report by the Tobacco Advisory Group of the Royal College of Physicians. London: RCP: Royal College of Physicians; 2007. Available from: https://www.rcplondon.ac.uk/publications/harm-reduction-nicotine-addiction.

284. National Institute for Health and Care Excellence. Smoking: harm reduction 2013. Available from: https://www.nice.org.uk/guidance/ph45/resources/smoking-harm-reduction-pdf-1996359619525.

285. Royal College of Physicians. RCP statement on e-cigarettes 2014. Available from: https://www.rcplondon.ac.uk/news/rcp-statement-e-cigarettes.

286. Australian Government Department of Health. National Drug Strategy 2017-2026 2017. Available from: https://www.health.gov.au/sites/default/files/national-drug-strategy-2017-2026_1.pdf.

287. Redmond H. The war on nicotine pits prejudice against Public Health. In Filter magazine 2018. Available from: https://filtermag.org/2018/09/25/the-war-on-nicotine/.

288. Warner KE. How to Think - Not Feel - about Tobacco Harm Reduction. *Nicotine Tob Res*. 2018

289. MacCoun RJ. Moral Outrage and Opposition to Harm Reduction. *Crim Law and Philos*. 2012 https://link.springer.com/article/10.1007/s11572-012-9154-0

290. McDonald CF et al. Electronic cigarettes: A position statement from the Thoracic Society of Australia and New Zealand. *Respirology*. 2020

291. Bates C. Understanding the war on vaping. In: The Tobacco Reporter. 2021. Available from: https://tobaccoreporter.com/2021/03/01/innovation-and-its-enemies/.

292. Mendelsohn CP. How opponents of vaping aid and abet Big Tobacco 2019. Available from: https://colinmendelsohn.com.au/wp-content/uploads/2020/01/How-opponents-of-vaping-aid-and-abet-Big-Tobacco.-The-Spectator.-Jan-2020.pdf.

293. Phillips CV. Why is there anti-THR? (3) Anti-tobacco extremism 2015. Available from: https://antithrlies.com/2015/07/24/why-is-there-anti-thr-3-anti-tobacco-extremism/.

294. Phillips CV. Why is there anti-THR? "Not Invented Here" syndrome 2015. Available from: https://antithrlies.com/2015/07/22/why-is-there-anti-thr-2-not-invented-here-syndrome/.

295. Sutherland R. Alchemy: The Surprising Power of Ideas That Don't Make Sense: WH Allen; 2019.

296. Tyndall M. Twitter post on tobacco control advocates and vaping 2021. Available from: https://twitter.com/DrMtyndall/status/1422636862666158083.

297. Newman J. Evidence-based policy or risk minimisation? The regulation of e-cigarettes in Australia. *Evidence & Policy*. 2019

298. Allsop S. Swimming with crocodiles: Lessons learned from 40 years of trying to influence policy 2020. Available from: https://ndarc.med.unsw.edu.au/resource/swimming-crocodiles-lessons-learned-40-years-trying-influence-policy.

299. Psychology Today. Groupthink 2019. Available from: https://www.psychologytoday.com/au/basics/groupthink.

300. Kahan DM. Why Smart People Are Vulnerable to Putting Tribe Before Truth. In: Scientific American blog 2018. Available from: https://blogs.scientificamerican.com/observations/why-smart-people-are-vulnerable-to-puttingtribe-before-truth/.

301. Juma C. Innovation and Its Enemies: Why People Resist New Technologies: Oxford University Press; 2016.

302. Commonwealth of Australia. Budget Strategy and Outlook Budget Paper No. 1, 2019-20 2020. Available from: https://www.budget.gov.au/2019-20/content/bp1/download/bp1.pdf.

303. Phillips CV. Why is there anti-THR? (4) Money, money, money 2015. Available from: https://antithrlies.com/2015/07/29/why-is-there-anti-thr-4-money-money-money/.

304. Mendelsohn CP. Tobacco tax rise exploits and punishes addicted smokers. In: news.com.au. 2017. Available from: https://www.news.com.au/lifestyle/health/health-problems/colin-mendelsohn-writes-tobacco-tax-rise-exploits-and-punishes-addicted-smokers/news-story/85537567d4893adf18f47a666df5d33a.

305. Public Health Law Centre - Mitchell Hamline School of Law. The Master Settlement: an overview 2019. Available from: https://www.publichealthlawcenter.org/sites/default/files/resources/MSA-Overview-2019.pdf.

306. Bates C. Holding the Bloomberg anti-vaping propaganda complex to account. The Counterfactual 2021. Available from: https://www.clivebates.com/holding-the-bloomberg-anti-vaping-propaganda-complex-to-account/#S13.

307. Oreskes N et al. Merchants of Doubt: Bloomsbury Press; 2010.

308. Brown and Williamson. Smoking and Health Proposal. Truth Tobacco Industry Documents. 1969. Available from: https://www.industrydocuments.ucsf.edu/tobacco/docs/#id=psdw0147.

309. Australian Tobacco Harm Reduction Association. An update on the lung disease outbreak in the US 2019. Available from: https://www.athra.org.au/blog/2019/09/07/an-update-of-the-lung-disease-outbreak-in-the-us/.

310. Australian Government Department of Health. E-cigarettes linked to severe lung illness 2019. Available from: https://www.health.gov.au/news/e-cigarettes-linked-to-severe-lung-illness.

311. Australian Tobacco Harm Reduction Association. Government officials misleading the Australian public on vaping needs to end 2019. Available from: https://www.athra.org.au/blog/2019/09/18/government-officials-misleading-the-australian-public-on-vaping-needs-to-end/.

312. Knott M. "Canary in the coal mine": US e-cigarette lung disease epidemic a worry: expert 2019. Available from: https://www.smh.com.au/world/north-america/canary-in-the-coal-mine-us-e-cigarette-lung-disease-epidemic-a-worry-expert-20190907-p52oye.html.

313. Tattan-Birch H et al. Association of the US Outbreak of Vaping-Associated Lung Injury With Perceived Harm of e-Cigarettes Compared With Cigarettes. *JAMA Netw Open*. 2020

314. Dave MD et al. News that takes your breath away: risk perceptions during an outbreak of vaping-related lung injuries. NBER Working Paper Series 2020. Available from: https://www.nber.org/papers/w26977#fromrss.

315. Redmond H. Anti-Vaping Zealots Find Opportunity in the Pandemic. In: Filter 2020. Available from: https://filtermag.org/anti-vaping-zealots-find-opportunity-in-the-pandemic/.

316. Victoria State Government Health and Human Services. Smoking and e-cigarette use. Coronavirus (COVID-19) 2020. Available from: https://www.dhhs.vic.gov.au/smoking-and-e-cigarette-use.

317. Gaiha SM et al. Association Between Youth Smoking, Electronic Cigarette Use, and COVID-19. *J Adolesc Health*. 2020

318. Channel 7 news. Young vapers more likely to get COVID-19 2020. Available from: https://7news.com.au/travel/coronavirus/young-vapers-more-likely-to-get-covid-19-c-1233383.

319. Bates C. Devastating post-publication peer reviews but the paper, PR and politics remain untouched 2020. Available from: https://pubpeer.com/publications/CEB008 BBD48F89272321EB50092793#7.

320. Farsalinos K et al. E-Cigarette Use and COVID-19: Questioning Data Reliability. *J Adolesc Health*. 2021

321. Kale D et al. Associations between vaping and Covid-19: Cross-sectional findings from the HEBECO study. *Drug Alcohol Depend*. 2021

322. Sussman RA et al. Aerial Transmission of the SARS-CoV-2 Virus through Environmental E-Cigarette Aerosols: Implications for Public Policies. *Int J Environ Res Public Health*. 2021

323. Chen J et al. A Comparative Health Risk Assessment of Electronic Cigarettes and Conventional Cigarettes. *Int J Environ Res Public Health*. 2017

324. McKee M et al. E-cigarettes should be regulated. *Med J Aust*. 2016

325. Hall B. Vaping likely to be banned in Melbourne CBD's smoke-free zones. In The Age. 2020. Available from: https://www.theage.com.au/politics/victoria/vaping-likely-to-be-banned-in-cbd-smoke-free-zones-20200727-p55fvd.html.

326. Chapman S. Twelve myths about e-cigarettes that failed to impress the TGA. The Conversation. 2017. Available from: https://theconversation.com/twelve-myths-about-e-cigarettes-that-failed-to-impress-the-tga-72408.

327. Chapman S et al. Submission to The Standing Committee on Health, Aged Care and Sport on Electronic Cigarettes and Vapourisers. Submission 313) 2017. Available from:

https://www.aph.gov.au/Parliamentary_Business/Committees/House/Health_Aged_ Care_and_Sport/ElectronicCigarettes/Submissions.

328. Public Health England. A note of errors concerning the UK in previous evidence submissions to the Committee 2017. Available from: https://www.aph.gov.au/ Parliamentary_Business/Committees/House/Health_Aged_Care_and_Sport/ ElectronicCigarettes/Submissions.

329. Creighton A. Health trio accused of presenting 'factual errors' to e cig inquiry. The Weekend Australian 2017. Available from: https://www.theaustralian.com.au/ national-affairs/health/health-trio-accused-of-presenting-factual-errors-to-ecig-inquiry/news-story/c360953ae14744b6beafc965eb1aa292.

330. Chapman S et al. Public Submission to the Senate Select Committee on Tobacco Harm Reduction. Submission 195 2020. Available from: https://www.aph.gov. au/Parliamentary_Business/Committees/Senate/Tobacco_Harm_Reduction/ TobaccoHarmReduction/Submissions.

331. McNeill A. Additional Comment to the Australian Select Committee on Tobacco Harm Reduction. Response to submission 195 2020. Available from: https://www. aph.gov.au/Parliamentary_Business/Committees/Senate/Tobacco_Harm_Reduction/ TobaccoHarmReduction/Submissions.

332. Brooke M. Talking Point: Vaping can hook a new generation. In the Mercury, Tasmania (print edition) 29 February 2020.

333. Australian Tobacco Harm Reduction Association. Lung Foundation Australia claims vaping as harmful as smoking 2020. Available from: https://www.athra.org.au/ blog/2020/03/04/lung-foundation-australia-claims-vaping-as-harmful-as-smoking/.

334. Australian Tobacco Harm Reduction Association. Lung Foundation Australia continues to mislead the public about vaping 2020. Available from: https://www.athra.org.au/ blog/2020/09/17/lung-foundation-australia-continues-to-mislead-the-public-about-vaping/.

335. Australian Tobacco Harm Reduction Association. Cancer Council Australia and Heart Foundation misinformed on vaping 2020. Available from: https://www.athra.org.au/ blog/2020/10/26/cancer-council-australia-and-heart-foundation-misinformed-on-vaping/.

336. ABC Sunshine Coast. Interview with AMA President, Dr Tony Bartone 2018. Available from: http://www.abc.net.au/radio/sunshine/programs/mornings/mornings/9926410.

337. 6PR Radio Station. Interview with AMA President, Dr Omar Khorshid 2018. Available from: https://www.6pr.com.au/podcast/medicos-split-over-e-cigs/.

338. Australian Tobacco Harm Reduction Association. It is legal to import nicotine into Queensland. 2018 https://www.athra.org.au/blog/2018/07/09/it-is-legal-to-import-nicotine-into-queensland/

339. Australian Tobacco Harm Reduction Association. Queensland Health caught out in vaping bungle … again 2019. Available from: https://www.athra.org.au/blog/2019/01/17/queensland-health-caught-out-in-vaping-bungle-again/.

340. Mendelsohn C. Prohibition and Misinformation: Australia's Tobacco Harm Reduction Fail. In Filter magazine 2019. Available from: https://filtermag.org/prohibition-and-misinformation-australias-tobacco-harm-reduction-fail/.

341. Australian Tobacco Harm Reduction Association. ATHRA in strong disagreement with Andrew Forrest. 2018 https://www.athra.org.au/blog/2018/08/31/athra-in-strong-disagreement-with-andrew-forrest/

342. McCauley D. Vaping: a harmless alternative, or a dangerous gateway to smoking? In Sydney Morning Herald and The Age. 2020. Available from: https://www.smh.com.au/politics/federal/vaping-a-harmless-alternative-or-a-dangerous-gateway-to-smoking-20200702-p558e7.html.

343. Han E. Secret industry funding of doctor-led vaping lobby group laid bare. In Sydney Morning Herald. 2018. Available from: https://www.smh.com.au/healthcare/secret-industry-funding-of-doctor-led-vaping-lobby-group-laid-bare-20180823-p4zzc5.html.

344. Smith R. Time to assume that health research is fraudulent until proven otherwise? Blog in: British Medical Journal. 2021. Available from: https://blogs.bmj.com/bmj/2021/07/05/time-to-assume-that-health-research-is-fraudulent-until-proved-otherwise/.

345. Rodu B. NIH Funding Stifles Tobacco Harm Reduction Research and Support in Academia. In Tobacco Truth blog. 2015. Available from: https://rodutobaccotruth.blogspot.com/2015/02/nih-funding-stifles-tobacco-harm.html.

346. Gunther M. Here Comes Trouble: An Anti-Tobacco Hero's Complicated Legacy. In Undark. 2021. Available from: https://undark.org/2021/08/02/here-comes-trouble-anti-tobacco-heroes-legacy/.

347. Retraction to: Electronic Cigarette Use and Myocardial Infarction Among Adults in the US Population Assessment of Tobacco and Health. *J Am Heart Assoc.* 2020 https://www.ahajournals.org/doi/abs/10.1161/JAHA.119.014519

348. Britton AR. Vaping and lung disease. In: The Times 2019. Available from: https://www.thetimes.co.uk/edition/comment/times-letters-proposed-overhaul-of-defence-spending-xmm9hwd8m.

349. Jensen RP et al. Hidden formaldehyde in e-cigarette aerosols. *N Engl J Med.* 2015

350. Farsalinos KE et al. E-cigarettes emit very high formaldehyde levels only in conditions that are aversive to users: A replication study under verified realistic use conditions. *Food Chem Toxicol.* 2017

351. Allen JG et al. Flavoring Chemicals in E-Cigarettes: Diacetyl, 2,3-Pentanedione, and Acetoin in a Sample of 51 Products, Including Fruit-, Candy-, and Cocktail-Flavored E-Cigarettes. *Environ Health Perspect.* 2016

352. Chivers E et al. Nicotine and other potentially harmful compounds in "nicotine-free" e-cigarette liquids in Australia. *Medical Journal of Australia*. 2019 Available at: https://www.mja.com.au/journal/2019/210/3/nicotine-and-other-potentially-harmful-compounds-nicotine-free-e-cigarette

353. The Logic of Science. 5 simple chemistry facts that everyone should understand before talking about science 2015. Available from: https://thelogicofscience.com/2015/05/27/5-simple-chemistry-facts-that-everyone-should-understand-before-talking-about-science/amp/?__twitter_impression=true.

354. Ames BN et al. The causes and prevention of cancer: gaining perspective. *Environ Health Perspect*. 1997

355. Vlachopoulos C et al. Electronic Cigarette Smoking Increases Aortic Stiffness and Blood Pressure in Young Smokers. *J Am Coll Cardiol*. 2016

356. Science Media Centre U. Expert reaction to three conference papers on e-cigarettes 2017. Available from: https://www.sciencemediacentre.org/expert-reaction-to-three-conference-papers-on-e-cigarettes/.

357. Borwein J et al. Clearing up confusion between correlation and causation. The Conversation 2014. Available from: https://theconversation.com/clearing-up-confusion-between-correlation-and-causation-30761.

358. Alzahrani T et al. Association Between Electronic Cigarette Use and Myocardial Infarction. *Am J Prev Med*. 2018

359. Critcher CR et al. Re-examining the Association Between E-Cigarette Use and Myocardial Infarction: A Cautionary Tale. *Am J Prev Med*. 2021

360. Bonn SA. Moral panic: who benefits from public fear. In: Psychology Today 2015. Available from: https://www.psychologytoday.com/intl/blog/wicked-deeds/201507/moral-panic-who-benefits-public-fear.

361. Boeri M. Re-criminalizing cannabis is worse than 1930s 'reefer madness'. In: The Conversation. 2018 https://theconversation.com/re-criminalizing-cannabis-is-worse-than-1930s-reefer-madness-89821

362. Hansen J. Deadly warning over teens' obsession with vaping. In: Daily Telegraph. 2021 https://www.dailytelegraph.com.au/subscribe/news/1/?source Code=DTWEB_WRE170_a_GGL&dest=https%3A%2F%2Fwww.dailytelegraph.com.au%2Fnews%2Fnsw%2Fwarning-on-vape-pens-as-teen-nearly-dies-vaping-is-not-cool%2Fnews-story%2Ff27580aa3af1b3e364912b97d073db62&memtype=register ed&mode=premium

363. Benowitz NL. Seizures After Vaping Nicotine in Youth: A Canary or a Red Herring? *J Adolesc Health*. 2020

364. AOD Media Watch. Demonising vaping: The Tele and APC threaten public health. 2021 https://www.aodmediawatch.com.au/demonising-vaping/

365. Paine H. Sydney teen issues vape warning after being hospitalised. In Daily Telegraph 2021. Available from: https://www.news.com.au/lifestyle/health/health-problems/sydney-teen-issues-vape-warning-after-being-hospitalised/news-story/887a69741c4ef86191a3779ac816ad7a.

366. Mendelsohn CP. Misinformation about vaping will keep adults smoking. In Alcohol and Other Drugs Media Watch 2021. Available from: https://www.aodmediawatch.com.au/misinformation-about-vaping/.

367. Therapeutic Goods Administration. Poisons Standard June 2021 (SUSMP no.22). Federal Department of Health 2021. Available from: https://www.legislation.gov.au/Details/F2021L00650.

368. World Health Organisation. Constitution of the World Health Organisation 1946. Available from: https://www.who.int/about/who-we-are/constitution.

369. United Nations. Universal Declaration of Human Rights 1948. Available from: https://www.un.org/en/about-us/universal-declaration-of-human-rights.

370. Global Commission on Drug Policy. War on drugs. Report. 2011. Available from: http://www.globalcommissionondrugs.org/wp-content/themes/gcdp_v1/pdf/Global_Commission_Report_English.pdf.

371. Volkow ND et al. Drug use disorders: impact of a public health rather than a criminal justice approach. *World Psychiatry*. 2017

372. Parliament of Victoria. Law Reform Road and Community Safety Committee. Inquiry ito drug law reform 2018. Available from: https://www.parliament.vic.gov.au/images/stories/committees/lrrcsc/Drugs_/Report/LRRCSC_58-03_Full_Report_Text.pdf.

373. Wikipedia. Harm Principle 2021. Available from: https://en.wikipedia.org/wiki/Harm_principle.

374. Hutcheon S et al. Smoke and mirrors: The nanny state critics behind the vape debate. ABC Background Briefing. 2019. Available from: https://www.abc.net.au/news/2019-08-30/nanny-state-critics-behind-the-vaping-debate/11449806?nw=0.

375. Clarke P et al. Mortality by Commonwealth Electoral Divisions in Australia. Public Health Information Development Unit, Torrens University Australia and Centre for Health Policy, University of Melbourne 2016. Available from: https://mspgh.unimelb.edu.au/__data/assets/pdf_file/0020/2001746/Mortality-by-CED-in-Australia-Report-June-2016.pdf.

376. Bonevski B et al. No smoker left behind: it's time to tackle tobacco in Australian priority populations. *Med J Aust*. 2018

377. Marmot M et al. Fair Society Healthy Lives 2010. Available from: http://www.instituteofhealthequity.org/resources-reports/fair-society-healthy-lives-the-marmot-review.

378. Giovenco DP. Different Smokes for Different Folks? E-Cigarettes and Tobacco Disparities. *Am J Public Health*. 2019

379. Brown J et al. Quit success rates in England 2007-2017. *Smoking in Britain*. 2017 Available at: http://www.smokinginbritain.co.uk/read-paper/draft/8/Quit%20 success%20rates%20in%20England%202007-2017

380. Kock L et al. E-cigarette use in England 2014-17 as a function of socio-economic profile. *Addiction*. 2018

381. Thirlway F et al. Tobacco smoking and vulnerable groups: Overcoming the barriers to harm reduction. *Addict Behav*. 2019

382. Twyman L et al. Electronic Cigarettes: Awareness, Recent Use, and Attitudes Within a Sample of Socioeconomically Disadvantaged Australian Smokers. *Nicotine Tob Res*. 2016

383. Gartner C. The potential impact of vaporized nicotine products on vulnerable subpopulations. *Addiction*. 2016

384. Pulvers K et al. Effect of Pod e-Cigarettes vs Cigarettes on Carcinogen Exposure Among African American and Latinx Smokers: A Randomized Clinical Trial. *JAMA Netw Open*. 2020

385. Brose LS et al. Mental health and smoking cessation-a population survey in England. *BMC Med*. 2020

386. Hoek J et al. A qualitative analysis of low income smokers' responses to tobacco excise tax increases. *Int J Drug Policy*. 2016

387. Bates C. The principle of proportionality The Tobacco Reporter2019. Available from: https://tobaccoreporter.com/2018/12/01/the-principle-of-proportionality/.

388. Magnusson RS. Time to raise the minimum purchasing age for tobacco in Australia. *Med J Aust*. 2016

389. Leventhal AM et al. Flavored E-cigarette Use and Progression of Vaping in Adolescents. *Pediatrics*. 2019

390. Wellman RJ et al. Predictors of the Onset of Cigarette Smoking: A Systematic Review of Longitudinal Population-Based Studies in Youth. *Am J Prev Med*. 2016

391. Buckell J et al. Should flavours be banned in cigarettes and e-cigarettes? Evidence on adult smokers and recent quitters from a discrete choice experiment. *Tob Control*. 2018

392. Friedman AS. A Difference-in-Differences Analysis of Youth Smoking and a Ban on Sales of Flavored Tobacco Products in San Francisco, California. *JAMA Pediatr*. 2021 https://doi.org/10.1001/jamapediatrics.2021.0922

393. Liber A et al. Flavored E-Cigarette Sales in the United States Under Self-Regulation From January 2015 Through October 2019. *Am J Public Health*. 2020

394. European Tobacco Harm Reduction Advocates (ETHRA). The EU Nicotine Users Survey 2020. The EU residents report 2021. Available from: https://ethra.co/images/Report_ ETHRA_Survey_2020_EN.pdf.

395. Posner H et al. Reactions to sales restrictions on flavored vape products or all vape products among young adults in the US. *Nicotine Tob Res*. 2021

396. Aslani A et al. Design, formulation and evaluation of nicotine chewing gum. *Adv Biomed Res*. 2012

397. Karasz P. Two UK Hospitals Allow Vape Shops in Bid to Promote Smoking Ban. The New York Times 2019. Available from: https://www.nytimes.com/2019/07/10/world/europe/uk-hospitals-vaping-shops.html.

398. Burstyn I. Peering through the mist: systematic review of what the chemistry of contaminants in electronic cigarettes tells us about health risks. *BMC Public Health*. 2014

399. Public Health England. Use of e-cigarettes in public places and workplaces. Advice to inform evidence-based policy making. PHE publications gateway number: 2016129 2016. Available from: https://www.gov.uk/government/uploads/system/uploads/attachment_data/file/534586/PHE-advice-on-use-of-e-cigarettes-in-public-places-and-workplaces.PDF.

400. The Royal Australian & New Zealand College of Psychiatrists. E-cigarettes and vaporisers. Position statement 97 2018. Available from: https://www.ranzcp.org/News-policy/Policy-submissions-reports/Document-library/E-cigarettes-and-vaporisers.

401. Dave D et al. Does e-cigarette advertising encourage adult smokers to quit? *J Health Econ*. 2019

402. UK Advertising Code. UK Code of Non-Broadcast Advertising 2016. Available from: https://www.cap.org.uk/Advertising-Codes/Non-Broadcast/CodeItem. aspx?cscid=%7B49028fdc-fc22-4d8a-ba5b-ba7ccc3df99a%7D#.V83uWDU6x0x

403. Jawad M et al. Price elasticity of demand of non-cigarette tobacco products: a systematic review and meta-analysis. *Tob Control*. 2018

404. Gorini G et al. The Regulatory Environment and Cost of Electronic Cigarettes in Italy, 2014-2015, Influenced their Use for Quitting. *Nicotine Tob Res*. 2018

405. Saffer H et al. E-cigarettes and adult smoking: evidence from Minnesota. National Bureau of Economic Research 2019. Available from: https://www.nber.org/papers/w26589.

406. Pesko MF et al. The Effect of Prices on Youth Cigarette and E-cigarette Use: Economic Substitutes or Complements? National Bureau of Economic Research 2017. Available from: https://papers.ssrn.com/sol3/papers.cfm?abstract_id=3077468.

407. Medicines and Healthcare products Regulatory Agency UG. Yellow Card Scheme 2021. Available from: https://yellowcard.mhra.gov.uk/.

408. Australian Tobacco Harm Reduction Association. Regulation of nicotine e-liquids for vaping in Australia 2020. Available from: https://athra.org.au/wp-content/uploads/2020/10/ATHRA-Vaping-Discussion-Paper-2Nov2020.pdf.

409.   Bonokoski M. Health Canada coughs up counterintuitive vape policy. In Toronto Sun 2021.

410.   Wikipedia. Social movement 2021. Available from: https://en.wikipedia.org/wiki/Social_movement.

411.   Australian Tobacco Harm Reduction Association. Australia's ban on nicotine importation lifted...for now 2020. Available from: https://www.athra.org.au/blog/2020/06/27/australias-ban-on-nicotine-importation-blocked-for-now/.

412.   District Court of Wellington. Ministry of Health v Phillip Morris (New Zealand) Limited. Judgement of Judge PJ Butler. Available from: https://www.districtcourts.govt.nz/assets/unsecure/2018-03-27/4f5561bf77/2018-NZDC-4478-MOH-v-Morris.pdf.

413.   Quebec Superior Court. Quebec Vaping Association vs Attorney General of Quebec 2019.   Available   from: http://www.cqct.qc.ca/Documents_docs/DOCU_2019/DOCU_19_05_03_Jugement_CourSuperieure_AQV.pdf.

414.   Federal Office of Public Health Switzerland. Lifting of the ban on the sale of snus 2019. Available   from: https://www.bag.admin.ch/bag/fr/home/das-bag/aktuell/news/news-011-06-2019.html.

415.   Planck MK. Planck's principle. In: Wikipedia. Available from: https://en.wikipedia.org/wiki/Planck%27s_principle.

416.   Australian Tobacco Harm Reduction Association. Australian and New Zealand medical specialists announce support for vaping. 2020. Available from: https://www.athra.org.au/blog/2020/04/23/australian-and-new-zealand-medical-specialists-announce-support-for-vaping/.

417.   British Medical Association. E-cigarettes: Balancing risks and opportunities. 2017. Available   at: https://www.bma.org.uk/collective-voice/policy-and-research/public-and-population-health/tobacco/e-cigarettes

418.   Academie Nationale de Medicine. Vaping nicotine 2019. Available from: https://www.academie-medecine.fr/lacademie-nationale-de-medecine-rappelle-les-avantages-prouves-et-les-inconvenients-indument-allegues-de-la-cigarette-electronique-vaporette/.

419.   Thomas KH, Dalili MN, López-López JA, et al. Smoking cessation medicines and e-cigarettes: a systematic review, network meta-analysis and cost-effectiveness analysis. Health Technol Assess 2021; 25 (59): 1-224 2021/10/21

420.   Rauch J. The Constitution of Knowledge: A defense of Truth: Brookings Institution; 2021

INDEX

Milton Keynes UK
Ingram Content Group UK Ltd.
UKHW020306050823
426346UK00012B/150